Psychotherapeutic Approaches to Sexual Problems

An Essential Guide for
Mental Health Professionals

Psychotherapeutic Approaches to Sexual Problems

An Essential Guide for Mental Health Professionals

Stephen B. Levine, M.D.

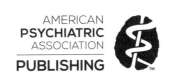

AMERICAN
PSYCHIATRIC
ASSOCIATION
PUBLISHING
™

Copyright © 2020 American Psychiatric Association Publishing

ALL RIGHTS RESERVED

Manufactured in the United States of America on acid-free paper
23 22 21 20 19   5 4 3 2 1

American Psychiatric Association Publishing
800 Maine Avenue SW, Suite 900
Washington, DC 20024-2812
www.appi.org

Library of Congress Cataloging-in-Publication Data
Names: Levine, Stephen B., author. | American Psychiatric Association, issuing body
Title: Psychotherapeutic approaches to sexual problems : an essential guide for mental health professionals / Stephen B. Levine.
Description: First edition. | Washington, D.C. : American Psychiatric Association Publishing, [2020] | Includes bibliographical references and index.
Identifiers: LCCN 2019031916 (print) | ISBN 9781615372836 (paperback : alk. paper) | ISBN 9781615372850 (ebook)
Subjects: MESH: Sexual Dysfunctions, Psychological—therapy | Psychotherapy—methods | Mental Health Services | Professional Practice
Classification: LCC RC557 (print) | LCC RC557 (ebook) | NLM WM 611 | DDC 616.85/830651—dc23
LC record available at https://lccn.loc.gov/2019031916
LC ebook record available at https://lccn.loc.gov/2019031917

British Library Cataloguing in Publication Data
A CIP record is available from the British Library.

With love and gratitude to my admirable daughter-in-law, Kathleen L. Levine, who is embarking on a career as a mental health professional

Contents

Preface

This book is primarily intended for new mental health professionals during or shortly after their final training experiences. Its purpose is to provide a sophisticated introduction to the sexual concerns of people who seek mental health care. The book addresses young professional readers from many backgrounds—psychiatry, psychology, social work, counseling, marriage and family therapy, nursing, and the clergy. I hope to interest readers from each of these groups to listen to their patients', clients', or congregation members' intimate relationship stories. While some patients will occasionally directly ask for help with their sexual concerns, most will first seek assistance with other problems. In doing so they often reveal aspects of their sexual and relational lives and share their perceived problems. Such revelations are often highly relevant to their presenting difficulties and ideally should be of interest to the therapist.

At every age and stage of the life cycle, sexuality can be fraught with concerns. There are times when a referral to a urologist, gynecologist, sex therapist, or gender specialist is useful. Many patients assume, however, that their mental health professional has an interest in, and knowledge about, sexual life because they realize that their sexual life is so subjectively psychological. They are dismayed when they are told such things as, "I don't specialize in sexual problems." When the psychosocial contributions to a problem are obvious to patients, they generally want to stay with their therapist. Referral may be experienced as a rejection and as an indication not to further discuss anything about their sexual lives with the therapist. In writing this book, I intended to minimize the frequency of such dampening responses. I thought I might best accomplish this goal by increasing my readers' comfort with the topic, stimulating their professional interest in this subject, and demonstrating how frequently people are disappointed in this aspect of their lives. An essential fund of knowledge is key in my estimation. When we begin to attend to patients' sexual disappointments and concerns—a process that is rarely available in our culture—our thoughtful interventions may prove to be of considerable help.

Sex is an important universal human functional activity for self-discovery, bonding, pleasure, nurturance, and reproduction. It poses at least three professional paradoxes. The first is that despite the fact that sexuality's importance to mental health has been recognized for over a century, training in the preclinical and clinical years tends to gloss over the topic. Trainees typically obtain few to no supervised experiences with sexual problems and, despite their personal interest in sexual matters, often steer clear of it in their clinical work. The second paradox is that sexual experiences are well known to consist of a finite set of behaviors. This gives the impression that it is a simple matter—that is, people have sexual intercourse. The more one studies the topic, however, the more individual the subjective and behavioral aspects are for each person and each couple. People may have several definable ways of having sex, but many come to not want to have any sexual activities or maintain highly restricted ones. In this way, sexuality is as individual as is the human face. Sexuality is both knowable at every stage of the life cycle and unique. The third paradox has to do with the diversity of human sexual experience. There is a both a wide range of behavioral and subjective expressions of sexual identity and a broad range in sexual functional capacities. This range in expressions and capacities is complicated further by the interaction of two people who may be incompatible in some ways as they interact to produce their coupled sexual lives. Despite this diversity of sexual lifestyles, interests, and capacities, many health professionals are given to simplifying this complexity so as to quickly treat problems. Erection problems: provide a drug. Gender dysphoria: encourage transition. Vaginismus: recommend dilators. Women's anorgasmia: masturbate. Such clinical reflexes based on the medicalization of sexuality do not reflect clinical sophistication. *Psychotherapeutic Approaches to Sexual Problems* is intended to demystify each of these paradoxes. I hope to provide readers with a conviction about the individuality of a person's sexual experience. In my view, this is vital to successful clinical treatment, a process that begins with the correct categorization of patients' stories.

I do not intend this book to be difficult to read, dry, or academic. I am content with not sharing all the known facts about a particular subject and the basis for how they became facts. The book is far more a supervisory guide to patients' stories, one that provides a useful perspective on them. If readers find this clinical introduction to be intellectually stimulating, there are many additional resources to continue their learning process. These include numerous textbooks, 86 specialty journals,[1] databases such as PubMed, and 31 national and international specialty organizations devoted to these problems.[2] The Internet provides easy access to many of these resources. Some of these are listed in the appendix to this book.

Because one person wrote this book, its text reflects his values, biases, limitations, strengths, clinical experiences, and understanding of the field.

There is no such thing as the final word or the best perspective on clinical sexuality. All people possess this multidimensional complexity; there are many lenses through which to view sexuality. Regardless of a person's gender identity, orientation, or sexual behavioral interest—that is, the individual's sexual identity—each person experiences an array of intensities of sexual desire, arousal, and orgasm. Sexual function is far more contextual and partner specific than is sexual identity. The study of sexual function applies to all people regardless of how they identify. As approximately 88% of the population labels themselves as heterosexual with a conventional form of gender identity and sexual behavioral patterns, much of this book addresses the problems they often encounter. But most of the discussions about sexual dysfunction apply to all people regardless of their sexual identities. As a significantly large minority of the population has differing sexual identities, their unique struggles are discussed as well.

It is hoped that this book will prove to be a trustworthy beginning to a lifelong educational process about individual sexualities. Perhaps one or more readers may be inspired to spend their careers helping others to learn about the ever-expanding topic of clinical sexuality.

Stephen B. Levine, M.D.
January 2019

References

1. Zucker KJ: Sex/gender/sexual science research 24/7. Arch Sex Behav 47(4):833–846, 2018
2. Wikipedia.org: List of sexology organizations. Available at: https://en.wikipedia.org/wiki/List_of_sexology_organizations. Accessed December 24, 2018.

1 | A Professional View of Sexual Life

As I welcome you to the fascinating but restricted realm of clinical sexuality, I am aware that you are already knowledgeable about your own sexuality. As you listen to the sexual problems of others, you will invariably reflect on your own development and current sexual life. Please do not fear this vital subjective process. A problem-free, concern-free, enjoyable sexual life is not a requirement to help others. All of us who aspire to sexual fulfillment are susceptible to disappointment. We face different challenges as our youth imperceptibly passes through various stages to old age. Sexual vulnerability always exists. As we allow ourselves to reflect on our own life, we come to see that sexual pleasure is rife with nuance, curiosity, possibility, and contradiction. I want to assure you that what you will be hearing from your patients will prove to be a major source of your expanding professional skills. Your patients will deepen your understanding of life processes and of yourself.

Respect for Privacy

Despite the numerous sexual images in modern culture, public references to sex and scandals, and commercial panaceas, the first important characteristic of any individual's sexuality is that it is private. Individuals guard their sexual lives with several distinct protective layers. We do not reveal everything to our partners. Partners keep their shared sexual behaviors to themselves. Individuals may not clearly tell themselves of their own desires. Children and adolescents keep their sexual thoughts and behaviors from their parents. It is our professional privilege that patients are willing to share aspects of their privacy so that we can help them. Session by session they reveal what they consider to be relevant to their problem. Privacy is so formidable a force,

1

however, that it is not realistic for us to expect that patients will ever reveal the entirety of their sexual lives to us. We are always working with limited information. Please do not be insulted; we aim for sufficient, not complete, knowledge.

Eroticism Versus Sexual Behaviors

An individual's sexuality involves both *eroticism*—the subjective experience of fantasy, desire, attraction, and preoccupation—and *sexual behaviors*. Professionally, we distinguish between eroticism and solo and partnered sexual behaviors, even though some of our colleagues and patients use these words as synonyms. Privacy envelops patients' eroticism and the identity of some of their past and present partners, and what behaviors they have engaged in. As a result of this natural guardedness, we content ourselves with what has been revealed and do not push patients beyond their comfort level. More details may or may not be forthcoming in future sessions.

Certain professional characteristics make it easier for patients to reveal their eroticism and sexual behaviors. Our interest, calm manner, knowledge of the problem, clarifying questions, and nonjudgmental attitude increase their confidence that it is safe to provide details to us. However, to the extent that we demonstrate the opposite traits—apparent anxiety, indifference, irrelevant questions, lack of information, and censoring responses—our chances for therapeutic success diminish. These positive professional characteristics are not different from the features required to deal skillfully with other mental health challenges. They are just more difficult to attain for young mental health professionals. There are several important reasons for this.

All of us have socially learned that eroticism and sexual behavior are matters so private that we should not ask such questions of a friend, relative, or acquaintance. We learn to talk around the subject unless the information is voluntarily shared. It is important to realize that our license—our culturally prescribed role as a therapist—enables us to be curious about this topic. Nonetheless, the layperson in a new professional role naturally avoids the subject and, when first confronted with a patient's sexual concern, may experience unease. Without in-depth discussions in seminars or in supervision, many young professionals will unfortunately avoid directly discussing sexual matters for the rest of their professional lives. They will use some justification, such as "Sexual problems are the result of other issues that I do focus on." The results are likely to be a failure to get to the heart of the patient's sexual experience and the attainment of a glancing view of their patients' sexuality. My colleagues and I have benefited from uncomfortable therapists in our community who do not feel equipped to respond to their patients' sexual concerns. They refer these patients to us. Sexual problems are too prevalent for this to be a good idea. The purpose of this book is to prevent professional avoidance of sexual concerns and to encourage therapists to try to personally be of assistance.

The Natural Voyeuristic Response

There is another reason why sexual topics create so much clinical discomfort. Each of us has a strong natural interest in the topic of sex, yet professionals sidestep the subject. Why? One way to find the answer is to consider the impact of movies on our subjective experiences. Scenes that are romantic, that suggest the imminence of lovemaking, or that explicitly display adults enjoying sex routinely sexually excite viewers. Our limbic systems respond with arousal when imagining or watching others behave sexually. This may occur even if we disapprove of what we are seeing. This voyeuristic response extends to reading about sex and listening to accounts of sexual behavior. Being slightly aroused, even transiently, in the context of clinical activities seems dangerous to many. Some clinicians think it forbidden. For instance, hearing about a patient's pleasures in oral-genital sex may immediately be arousing or take the professional to his or her own experiences. This may create arousal, disgust, or envy. We are human. What we listen to, we subjectively respond to. When we consider our private response to be unprofessional, we will find a way to avoid repeating the experience in the future.

What is forbidden, what is clearly unethical, are the behaviors that constitute the slippery slope to violation—the flirtations, compliments, and personal revelations. These behaviors typically precede sexual behavior with the patient. Sex with a patient is defined as the use of the patient's body for the professional's pleasure or the use of the patient's mind for the clinician's arousal. Thus, sex can occur without intercourse and can include sharing erotic fantasies about each other. We are not going to confuse such professional sexual boundary violations, however, with our private transient experiences of arousal and our private personal comparisons with what the patients are reporting. Violation of the sanctity of the professional relationship is light-years away from these ordinary momentary subjective experiences when trying to improve a patient's sexual life. The confusion of these two phenomena creates the obstacle to future effective clinical work with sexual problems.

Eroticism and the Limitation of Clinical Work

Much of conscious life about sexuality does not involve behavior. It involves fleeting thoughts and brief waves of feeling. These subjective erotic processes are far more common in adolescence and young adulthood but are part of most people's lives throughout the life cycle, particularly when individuals are physically well and not overwhelmed by some dilemma. When sharing eroticism, patients can only make general summary statements about what is or what is not occurring in their minds about themselves and others. The inherent limitations in the accuracy of patient summaries of their erotic experiences derive from how difficult it is to be a reliable narrator of this mental arena. Their need for privacy, embarrassment, fear of your disapproval, and unexpected spontaneous mental events contribute to this. We have discovered, for instance, that many women who sought help for low or absent sexual desire had some manifestations of sexual desire. It may have been that their summary was correct about the paucity of their desire, or that desire reappeared during our work together in research or in therapy, or that they understood desire to be for their partner rather than for anyone in particular. We have also learned that men may complain of erectile problems when, in fact, they have rapid uncontrollable ejaculation, or complain that they have premature ejaculation when, in fact, they have erectile dysfunction, or both. We need to accept that patients tell us what they are able to share, and it is our responsibility to clarify their complaint more accurately.

We Are Part of History

The work that we are undertaking to better understand how to assist patients in this arena of life has its roots in the earliest of medical writings.[1] In every era, professional writings begin with classification, move on to theories of causation, and end with therapeutic suggestions. These processes reflect cultural understandings of illness in that period.[2] In the last 60 years we have witnessed a progression from a simple Freudian classification of impotence and frigidity, to Masters and Johnson's expanded list of three sexual dysfunctions for each sex, to the further expanded nosology in DSM-5, which will soon be challenged by the yet unfinished schema in ICD-11. The sexuality patterns that we will be considering are those that are brought to our clinical attention, only some of which can be found in a committee-approved nosological schema.

The Natural Division

Health and disorder perspectives on the sexual universe naturally divide into two broad dimensions: sexual identity and sexual function. Psychiatry, psychology, and the numerous master's degree–prepared fields of psychotherapy usually begin the education of their students with the designated problems in these two dimensions because those fields were created to solve them. Wide variations in each of these major categories of sexuality are more apparent now than ever before in history; diversity is also seen in the behaviors that individuals engage in.[3] In recent decades mental health professionals are pathologizing less and understanding more. This alone represents cultural progress.

Sexual identity has three components: gender identity, orientation, and intention (see Chapter 7 for further discussion). Passionate politics surround the variations in these components as different stakeholders defend or condemn those with nonconforming gender identities, homosexual interests and behaviors, and unconventional or paraphilic desires and behaviors. We mental health professionals are not expected to be a part of those who condemn because we are devoted to helping. In the past we have been condemnatory, most vociferously, about homosexual lives.[4] Groups of people who in the past found themselves in classification systems of mental disorders are today more neutrally referred to as sexual minority members or their interests and desires are subsumed under the umbrella of sexual diversity.

Sexual function has four components: desire, arousal, penetration, and orgasm. Their problematic aspects are classified by genital anatomy. Male DSM-5 diagnoses are male hypoactive sexual desire disorder, erectile disorder, premature (early) ejaculation, and delayed ejaculation. Female DSM-5 diagnoses are female sexual interest/arousal disorder, female orgasmic disorder (anorgasmia), and genito-pelvic pain/penetration disorder. Both men and women have substance/medication-induced problems. DSM-5 creates other specified and unspecified categories for other patterns. Do not be misled by the terms *male* and *female* in these headings. Gender-nonconforming individuals may also qualify for these DSM-5 sexual dysfunction diagnoses.

Where Do We Learn About the Sources of Sexual Problems?

Movies, television, fiction, biography, newspapers, magazines, talks with friends, watching dramas unfold in our family and the families of our friends, and self-knowledge all contribute to what we know about the causes of personal and interpersonal dilemmas that may limit sexual life. Some of these are accurate illustrations of how people suffer, and even though they may not deal with sexual identity and function directly, people intuit how sexual life may be affected. We also learn about sexual life from our knowledge of medicine, where sexually transmitted diseases, pregnancy and its complications, gynecological and urological diseases, and organ system failures interfere with self-concepts, pleasure, and sexual capacities. And, depending on our knowledge of different cultures, we may realize how the ideas unique to these cultures may facilitate or constrain sexual development. All of us have ideas about what influences sexual life. One of the things that limit our understanding of these influences is the enormous variation in every aspect of sexuality.

The questions for professionals are 1) Do we know something that observant laypersons do not know? 2) Do we have esoteric information or a frame of understanding that is more or less unique to us? 3) To what extent can clinical science help us? and 4) Is the knowledge generated by clinical science useful to the process of helping? I will provide you with my answers to these four closely related questions in Chapter 10.

How Individuals Become Patients

We live our lives. At times, our feelings and behaviors create situations that we cannot master. This does not cause most people to seek assistance from a mental health professional. At times, others tell individuals that they need professional assistance. Even this does not necessarily result in their seeking our assistance. At best about half of physician referrals to a mental health professional are acted on and often not immediately. Numerous studies have illustrated that most people with "mental disorders" do not seek mental health care and that most people with sexual difficulties do not directly ask for help.[5] We assume that those who do arrive for care inform us of the sexual vulnerabilities of the population who do not seek care. But we can never be sure how great a public health problem our patients' concerns represent. My synthesis is that my patients represent the very tip of the iceberg of prevalence.

Happy, sexually well-adjusted, fulfilled people generally do not seek our services. Most seek us out in crisis or after bearing the weight of a serious dilemma for a long period of time. Three avenues to care provide us with our clinical experiences: 1) an individual or couple arrives with a chief complaint of a sexual identity or a sexual function concern; 2) an individual seeks treatment for another psychiatric problem and eventually discusses her sexual problem; or 3) an institution such as a hospital, school, corporation, or religious organization, or a lawyer or judge, remands a person for evaluation after his sexual behavior offended the institution's or society's values.

These pathways have taught us that there are recurring sexual patterns that are not well characterized in any nosology. These include the unconsummated marriage; a couple's abandonment of sexual behavior; unreliable sexual function during infertility treatment; sexual aversion; orgasm with diminished pleasure; sexual addiction; sex crimes; persistent genital arousal; and individuals who become physically ill following orgasm. Even this list, however, does not capture the vital life-diminishing problems of infidelity, jealousy, pornography dependence, the love-lust split, and the impact of physical illness, including that related to a sexually transmissible infection. Nor does it capture a variety of context-specific subjective concerns that are impossible to completely list.[6] Here are only a few: Can I sustain love for any partner? When should I fake orgasm? What will menopause do to me? How long will my waning potency last? Why can't I enjoy this? Am I gay? Am I trans? Interest in clinical sexuality exposes the clinician to all the processes of life. One cannot listen to sexual stories from patients without eventually coming to appreciating this.

Impacts Working With Sexual Problems Can Have on You

This book is not intended to train you as a sex specialist. It is intended to prepare you to be interested and helpful in your specific work setting, which will vary considerably from reader to reader. As long as you are open to listening to patients' concerns, you may encounter all of the patterns mentioned in the previous section. Although you will not be able to resolve all of them, your efforts to understand can be helpful. Your rewards for trying will often be patient respect, gratitude, and future referrals.

Working with patients' sexual concerns will show you that sexuality is not simply about sex. The topic is actually about the unfolding of the individual self, the capacity to give and receive pleasure, the ability to be psychologically intimate, the capacity to love and to be loved, and the ability to manage the expected and unexpected changes that occur throughout adulthood. You will soon begin to have convictions about what shapes a person's fate. With just a little experience you will be able to get to the heart of a clinical situation more efficiently. You may realize the profound hopes for a better life that patients have during their work with you. You may find that your sexual life improves as a result of your changing perspectives. And you will remain professionally humbled by the fact that although you can help many, there is so much that you cannot positively influence. A sexuality focus is just one of many clinical pathways to these professional goals, but since every patient you will ever work with will have a sexuality, you are bound to discover a sexual universe that is well beyond your current understanding. You need only remain a respectful, curious student who is committed to assist, no matter your age, gender, orientation, or preferred ideology.

References

1.   Berry M: The history and evolution of sex therapy and its relationship to psychoanalysis. International Journal of Psychoanalytic Studies 10(1):53–74, 2013
2   Jones DP: The burden of disease and the changing task of medicine. N Engl J Med 366(25):2333–2338, 2012
3.   Herbenick D, Bowling J, Fu TJ, et al: Sexual diversity in the United States: results from a nationally representative probability sample of adult women and men. PLoS One July 20;12(7):e0181198, 2017
4.   Committee on Human Sexuality of the Group for the Advancement of Psychiatry: Homosexuality and the Mental Health Professions: The Impact of Bias. Report 144. Hillsdale, NJ, Analytic Press, 2000
5.   March D, Oppenheimer DM: Social disorder and diagnostic order: the US Mental Hygiene Movement, the Midtown Manhattan study and the development of psychiatric epidemiology in the 20th century. Int J Epidemiol 43(suppl 1):i29–i42, 2014
6.   Levine SB: Towards a compendium of the psychopathologies of love. Arch Sex Behav 43(1):213–220, 2013

2 | The Simple Male Dysfunction

Three Fundamental Notions Pertaining to All the Dysfunctions

Before we get to premature ejaculation, which is the most straightforward male sexual dysfunction, I need to share some basic information about the complex sources of any sexual dysfunction, including premature ejaculation. Four bedrock forces continually shape our sexual lives. Each of these influences is subtly ever changing throughout life.

1. The body's capacities
2. The individual's unique past and current psychology
3. The nature of the relationship with the partner
4. The person's culture

The appreciation of this concept alone—four interacting shaping forces—should be sufficient to keep clinicians and researchers humble.

Two other essential perspectives are needed to prepare for our work. Our thinking about sexual problems is organized by

1. *Biological sex*—that is, does this body possess anatomic and physiological femaleness or maleness?
2. *Stage in the life cycle that the patient occupies*. I prefer this designation to the use of the term *age*.

These factors are relevant when we consider the biology and psychology of sexual capacity, motivations for sexual behavior, vulnerability to sexual concerns, and meanings of relationship processes.

A third fundamental perspective is articulated by the question "Who is this person?" The answer can yield a far more erudite perception of the patient than sex and stage in life. The answer will rest on everything that you know as a person and everything you have learned as a mental health professional. We are trained to begin our assessments and our formal case presentations with identifying information (e.g., "Dr. M is a 6′6″ thin retired 55-year-old general surgeon, recently divorced father of a son, age 11 years, and a daughter, age 14 months"). Each of the specifying words in such a sentence prepares our minds to listen intently to what the patient will share with us. The better we accurately characterize the patient, the better our chances will be of forming a good therapeutic alliance, tuning into the patient's needs, and grasping how those four bedrock forces have contributed to his chief complaint and underlying sexual difficulty.

From Etiology to Pathogenesis to Pathways

I try not to use the term *etiology* for psychiatric or sexual problems unless the immediate precipitants are conspicuous and consistent from one person to the next. Our mental health fields still appropriate this historic infectious disease model of causality despite our absolute failure to scientifically assign a single cause to any of our major conditions.[1] Sometimes we come close, as in postcombat posttraumatic stress disorder or intense prolonged grief after a death of a spouse, but modern authors typically characterize etiology of DSM-5 disorders as multifactorial, as explained by environment-gene interaction, as neurobiological, as having temperamental predisposition, or as having 40% genetic variance. That there are genetic influences on mental disorders is a widely accepted fact limited by the observation that the same genes predispose to multiple diagnoses. Such general statements, although soothing to our intellect, are very different than etiological formulations from a half century ago. Every era seems to create its separate notions of etiology. I submit that few of them help us with our daily work of trying to improve patients' lives.

I prefer to discuss the origins of sexual problems in terms of the apparent pathways that led to the issue at hand. Sometimes I refer to this as *pathogenesis*, but that word connotes a more biological mechanism than, for instance, how the discovery of betrayal rearranges the psyche and creates sexual aversion. The first syllable in pathogenesis implies an abnormal process. So I generally speak of the pathways to the problem, leaving room for factors that may be inherent in the patient or factors originating from outside the patient. Sometimes it is normal to be "abnormal"—that is, to experience a loss of all sexual interest after the death of a beloved partner.

My quest to understand the sources of sexual problems has been assisted by my experiences at interdisciplinary meetings of those interested in sexual medicine, sexology, and sex therapy. These professionals include urologists, gynecologists, internists, psychologists, advanced practice nurses, physical therapists, pharmacological researchers, sex therapists, and other mental health professionals who share an interest in helping patients with their sexual lives. It is a bit of a Tower of Babel listening to diverse professionals classify problems, discuss etiology, and offer treatments. This has taught me that every specialty simplifies the actual complexity of sexual problems. Various medical specialists offer different treatments. To overgeneralize: gynecologists offer hormones, urologists provide surgery and medications, primary care doctors and psychiatrists change medications, psychologists offer psychotherapy, sex therapists offer intimate exercises, physical therapists offer pelvic floor retraining, and pharmacological researchers propose new medications. All of us make use of the significant placebo response, which, while wonderful in its power to cause improvement, can be clinically misleading. It often seems that theories of causality follow from the treatments that are being offered. For example, when flibanserin was approved for menstruating women's loss of sexual desire, the idea was promulgated that the affected woman had a biochemical brain-based problem that the medication improved. Some practitioners who advocate for puberty suppression for trans children promulgate the idea that gender dysphoria is neurologically determined.

Mental health professionals are limited by our methods—listening, discussing, educating, synthesizing, and suggesting. Physicians dealing with anatomy and physiology often see problems that are invisible to us—atrophic vulvovaginitis, pelvic misalignment, and hip labrum tears. There is no reason for mental health professionals to feel inferior because of our lack of access to the body's subtle ailments or to feel superior because of our capacities to consider the psychosocial contributions over time. We, too, are but one type of professional in a long chain of those who may assist.

Actual progress is made in two related ways: initially illuminating the pathways to the problem or ameliorating the problem and working backward to explain its mechanism. Either way, we come to better understand how the problem develops. When the origins of problems are not well understood, treatments multiply, but they disappear quickly over time. When the origins are defined, treatments are few and persist. Testosterone for women complaining of low sexual desire now seems passé.[2] The phosphodiesterase-5 (PDE-5) inhibitor medications have been used effectively for men with unreliable erections for more than two decades. We can now explain how these medications help sexually anxious men through vascular and psychological mechanisms.[3]

One of the many limitations of clinical sexuality is our professional inability to demarcate the boundaries between disorder and the broad range of normal experience.[4] Is a woman's rate of orgasmic attainment with a partner normal at 66% and abnormal at 33%? Is time to ejaculation after penetration normal if it is 75 seconds and abnormal if it is 50 seconds? Nosology committees arbitrarily answer these questions when they define a disorder, but their criteria do not determine who seeks help for anorgasmia or rapid ejaculation.

What to Do

Our work quickly goes beyond diagnostic criteria in trying to understand how the presenting issue came to be defined by the patient or couple as a problem. When we learn that a man has been a rapid ejaculator all his life and that he arrives for help now because his wife no longer wants to have sex and he suspects she has someone else in her life, we realize that we are being asked to take into consideration something beyond the medication treatment of his DSM-5 diagnosis. There are pathways to symptoms and there are consequences of symptoms. Patients bring both to us. Our response to patients is expected to vary case by case, but generally these are the steps we try to follow.

1. Assign a diagnostic category to the nature of the patient's problem. Is this a sexual identity or sexual dysfunction issue or both?
2. Characterize the symptom pattern as lifelong, acquired, situation specific, or generalized to all sexual opportunities. This is crucial in directing our further inquiries.
3. Determine why the person is seeking help at this time. Failure to do this will likely significantly delay the professional from getting to the heart of the matter.
4. Organize the pathways to the problem in the light of three types of factors:
   a. Those that seem to have originally precipitated the symptom
   b. Those that seem to maintain the symptom
   c. Those that seem to have predisposed the person to the symptom or to the response to the symptom

Sensuality and Performance Anxiety

Satisfying functional sex requires the abandonment of ordinary daily preoccupations and the substitution of a focus on bodily sensations. This is typically what occurs early in foreplay. Sensuality is not how a person looks. It is what a person is capable of doing and feeling during sex. A healthy muscular young man with a six-pack abdomen and a handsome face, attractive as he may be to many, is not necessarily a sensual person. Sensuality has two aspects. The readily appreciated one is the capacity to experience the preoccupying sensations of a kiss, lick, a touch, and a breast or genital caress and of penetration. Its more subtle aspect is the person's interest in transporting the partner to this realm where pleasure at the skin and mucus membranes predominates. Individuals may be better at one aspect of sensuality than another. They may prefer to provide, or they may prefer to receive, or ideally they easily can slip from giving to receiving and from receiving to giving. Even quick-to-intercourse sex can be sensuous, although what is usually meant by sensuous sex requires more time to give up ordinary daily concerns to the intense focus on what is being touched.

The pathway to all the sexual dysfunctions involves subtle obstacles to attaining a sensuous state. Once a dysfunctional symptom becomes established, it adds to the lack of sensuality because the person develops performance anxiety. Originally described as a characteristic of men with erection problems, performance anxiety was understood to be the vigilant preoccupation with how firm the erection was from moment to moment during foreplay culminating in a dread of failure in the vagina.[5] A man's performance anxiety could readily be communicated to his partner, inducing the partner's inability to become sensuous and aroused. But it is now apparent that men and women, regardless of their sexual dysfunction diagnosis, develop performance anxiety—that is, they become cognitively preoccupied with how they are doing or how they will feel a few minutes from now when intercourse or genital stimulation is attempted. This mental preoccupation prevents them from abandoning themselves to sensations from touch. Arousal derives from sensuality; anxiety diminishes the capacity to attend to the skin and the subtle cues from how it is being touched.

Premature or Rapid Ejaculation

The usual symptom pattern of this dysfunction is that it has been apparent from the beginning of partner sexual life (i.e., "lifelong"). The heterosexual man[*] has always found that intercourse quickly terminates his arousal

---

[*]There is no reason to assume that men who have sex with men are not concerned with patterns of rapid ejaculation. In fact, surveys have indicated a similar frequency of premature ejaculation (variously defined).[6] Nonetheless, almost the entire literature of premature ejaculation involves heterosexual men with women.

sooner than he desires, without the sense that he can control when orgasm occurs. Orgasm happens to him; he plays no role in inducing it. He senses himself to be sexually too excitable. While this may involve fellatio, if he even allows it, the crescendo to orgasm is typically most evident in the vagina.

This pattern is reported to be responsive to the use of any number of serotonergic medications, tramadol, topical anesthetics, and PDE-5 inhibitors, making the complaint treatable by any physician. This has led to the idea that there is something biologically different in these men.[7] It seems that their sensations from sexual stimulation of any part of their body, but particularly the penis, trigger orgasm much faster than the average man with the same degree of sexual experience. Almost all teenagers have unexpectedly reached orgasm during their first intimate experiences—for instance, first tongue-to-tongue exchange or first caress of the clothed pelvis. We might say arousal was overwhelming. The vast majority of young men do not continue to be this overpowered by arousal. With subsequent encounters, their nervous systems respond differently. However, it appears that 2%–4% of men continue to be overwhelmed as sexual intimacy continues over time (as measured with a stopwatch).[8] This figure is not consistently found. It has been estimated to be about 18% in Italy, for example (as measured by questionnaires).[9] There is no single character trait found among these men, who generally are physically and mentally perceived to be normal. This adds to the idea that they share a neurophysiological mechanism that the majority of men do not have. Today, this is thought to involve serotonin physiology.

I am delighted to alleviate the pattern, and the anxiety and disappointment that accompany it, with medication. But I see additional opportunities for mental health professionals to help. Culture infiltrates the bedroom in terms of shaping expectations for male and female roles and capacities. It is ironic that women who are readily aroused during sexual behavior—those who can quickly attain orgasm by hand, mouth, or penile insertion—are viewed as sexually competent and proudly treasured by themselves and their partners. Yet men who are readily aroused to orgasm may experience psychological and interpersonal distress.

One of the things that a mental health professional is called upon to do is to declare what is not the disorder of premature ejaculation. Much rapid ejaculation frequently occurs during adolescents' or young adults' first opportunities for intercourse, fellatio, or penile caressing with a new partner. It often occurs among partnered heterosexual men when sex resumes after a long absence. Rapid ejaculation may be expected to recur at the start of a new sexual relationship anytime during middle or older age. Men and their wise partners change these patterns by frequently repeating the sexual behavior. The partner's sensual ministrations and her orifices soon excite to the point of a plateau of arousal without the dreaded crescendo to orgasm. If he occasionally thereafter quickly reaches orgasm, the couple merely think it is just part of the wide variation in sexual experience brought about by changing neural and psychological sensitivities. We must recognize such circumstances so that the man who wrongly diagnoses himself with premature ejaculation obtains our thoughtful further inquiry.

> A single 24-year-old computer programmer sought help for premature ejaculation, saying that he can only last 4–6 minutes with his girlfriend of 4 months. Her previous boyfriend could provide twice as much time during intercourse, she told him. His two prior partners had never brought up the topic. As additional evidence of his dysfunctional state, he spoke of repeatedly witnessing men last much longer times in pornography. Several friends and acquaintances had commented on their intercourse prowess.

Despite the name of the disorder, time in the vagina alone is not an adequate criterion for the diagnosis. Many sensuous couples slowly and skillfully build their arousal together and connect their genitals only at a high level of mutual excitement. His rapidly attained orgasm often is the trigger for his partner's. The men we usually get to see are those whose lifelong patterns are to ejaculate within a minute of entering the vagina (the current diagnostic time criterion). When the man is more carefully questioned, when the partner is asked, or when seconds to ejaculation after vaginal entry are timed with a stopwatch, we learn that with few exceptions, the majority of men ejaculate within 30 seconds, depriving the partner of the sensuous experience of longer intercourse. So, of course, time is important. Couples may learn to adapt to this pattern by bringing the partner to orgasm by hand, mouth, or vibrator stimulation before intercourse. Other women adapt by reaching orgasm quickly during intercourse. Some men ignore their partners' needs and without much discussion just have intercourse. Resentful partners may refer to this as masturbating in their bodies. The men who come to us want to be more able providers of pleasure, so it is important they we tell them how to do that. I provide five ideas to them.

1. Stop saying, "I'm sorry!" "Dammit!" "Shit!" and so forth when you feel yourself about to come.
2. Instead, feel the pleasure of the orgasm and make the sounds of delight that naturally occur before and during orgasm. Do not silently come. Allow her to know you in this new way.
3. Feel all the contractions of orgasm over the next 25 seconds, not simply the first one that used to trigger your vocalized disappointment. Reversing these three patterns will quickly stop ruining the experience of orgasm

for you and your partner. The man immediately sees that these suggestions will enhance his and his partner's pleasure because orgasm can be
a positive reward for both of them. His orgasm can create a sense of closeness, which is no longer followed by self-derogation. "I'm sorry that I disappointed you. I'm such a loser" becomes "It was so wonderful to be inside
you."

4. Do not quickly withdraw from your partner's body after ejaculation. Wait
   until the detumescence is complete so that she can continue to feel you
   inside of her. She may be able to enjoy your increasingly soft penis for
   about 30 seconds. She does not necessarily need your erect penis to attain
   orgasm.

5. Stop thinking you have to bring her to orgasm through intercourse. You are
   just pressuring yourself into a greater degree of performance anxiety. Try
   to have intercourse with her on top in the following manner. Think of an-
   choring your erection in her body so that she can move slightly but firmly
   at her own pace in a head-to-toe direction against the anchor. Not only will
   this stimulate you less, she will arouse herself more, providing her with an
   opportunity to bring herself to orgasm. If she instead moves up and down
   on your penile shaft, she is generally going to induce your orgasm. There
   is no reason why she cannot use both movements, but this position is her
   opportunity to lead herself to greater arousal. Her orgasmic sounds may
   then induce your orgasm.

While discussing these points, I emphasize the need for the man to become
sensuous, and to put an end to his preventing his partner from trying to excite him. I tell him that the original therapy for this problem by Masters and
Johnson was to teach the couple how to make love without intercourse for
days before dealing directly with the rapidity of ejaculation. They were ex-
posing the man and his partner to more arousal. Their method was counter-
intuitive to their patients' reflexes to minimize their arousal. We no longer need
the 2 weeks of daily therapy that Masters and Johnson required to accomplish
the same goals, but we must understand these concepts and put them into play.

These ideas fill most men with a new hope for their future. They typically
say that they have never heard of these ideas before. They confess how embarrassed they have been to bring the subject up with anyone, including their
doctor and their partner. I give them 25 mg of clomipramine (Anafranil) to take
4 days in a row before they can expect a doubling of their time in the vagina.
If their sexual behaviors occur predictably—for example, on weekends—I have
them take 25 mg or 50 mg 4 days before sex. If sex occurs unpredictably, I
recommend taking the drug daily. Typically, there are no side effects at 25 mg,
but a slight headache and a tendency toward constipation may occur at 50

mg. Typically, 50 mg produces a longer capacity to be in the vagina than the beginning dose. The cholinergic side effects at 75 mg are usually too prominent to make this dosage useful, but an occasional man may require this much or more without bothersome side effects. Most men experience the return of their rapid ejaculation pattern when they stop the drug. Recently urologists in Korea demonstrated that this drug can be effectively used "on demand," 2–6 hours before intercourse.[10]

Many clinicians use other selective serotonin reuptake inhibitors (SSRIs), serotonin-norepinephrine reuptake inhibitors, or other medications for this purpose.[11] The PDE-5 inhibitors are expensive. The use of tramadol worries me because of the addiction potential of this mild opioid, and many patients have already tried a topical anesthetic.[12] I imagine that once a man discovers the positive impact of any of these drugs, he experiments with how to best use them. The problem is solved and the physician is no longer needed. I have a number of patients who have asked for their clomipramine to be renewed annually.

> A man with recently acquired erectile dysfunction regularly had rapid ejaculation during his 14 years of sexual experiences. My advice and clomipramine quickly helped him. We had a brief follow-up in 2 weeks. I said he could choose to take 50 mg as an experiment and gave him a 1-year prescription. Two months later he wrote that his wife was regularly orgasmic for the first time in her life.

But what do we do with the men like the one I briefly described who is concerned that his wife, who now refuses to have sex with him, is involved with another man? We discuss each of the topics in depth that he has highlighted. What is the basis of his thinking that there is another person involved with her? We inquire about what happened prior to her refusing to have sex. What did she say? What does he think caused her to abandon him sexually? What the patient and I are doing is ascertaining whether now is the time to treat his rapid ejaculation or whether we should work together to help him sort out his relationship status, alone or with his wife, before we deal with the rapid ejaculation pattern. This type of process cannot be expected to occur in a medical setting. He is fortunate that we are mental health professionals.

So, do men who regularly experience premature ejaculation and readily orgasmic women share rapid arousal to orgasm? In a sense, they do. But the women are not anxious, they are not strategizing, they are not repeating baseball scores, they are not monitoring their arousal in an attempt to attenuate it, and they are not masturbating to orgasm before sex. Rather, they love to be stimulated, look forward to it, and as a result love what their bodies can do for them. We are trying to get these men to better resemble these women.

Recently Acquired Rapid Ejaculation

Occasionally, you will encounter men with a new pattern of uncontrollable orgasm with a partner. Be glad. A man who never had this problem over many years develops it with the same partner or with a new partner after divorce or widowhood for a reason that you will eventually be able to define, even if he cannot initially identify the factor. The pattern just begs you to find the pathway to dysfunction. My first patient with this pattern developed it after his wife, who had become more obsessed with clothes and makeup as she was getting near menopause, was arrested for shoplifting. He then learned it was her third arrest. He was trying not to express the fullness of his anger at her. My second patient developed premature ejaculation after recovering from a myocardial infarction. He was trying to reassure himself of his potency but recognized he was afraid of dying during sex. I sent my third patient to a neurologist because he mentioned having abnormal sensations in his legs. The neurologist informed him that he had multiple sclerosis. My fourth patient developed it after he thought he had forgiven his wife for her recent affair. The three of us discussed "premature forgiveness."

It is a bit more difficult when a man develops rapid ejaculation for the first time with a new partner. You will ask open-endedly how she differs from his previous one. You will try to ascertain whether it is he who is putting pressure on himself to perform in some unrealistic manner or whether it is her expectations for long, hard intercourse that has put him in a state of sexual anxiety and dread of the next encounter. Before reaching for an SSRI-like drug, please be curious. Many of these men will have already taken a PDE-5 inhibitor, hoping to last longer on a second intercourse. I can think of no commonly used medications that cause this pattern, but, of course, we must consider diseases of the spinal cord and brain, which in some unknown way interfere with the processing of sensations. Unlike lifelong premature ejaculation, the time criterion for the acquired form is a decrease in former time in the vagina to 3 minutes or less.[13] In these cases, the time per se is not as crucial as the lost capacity.

The gender and sexual identities of therapists are far less important to the effective delivery of these ideas than the therapists' growing comfort with discussing these correctable patterns. Male professionals can be as initially uncomfortable as women. Some patients will remark that they prefer one gender or another, but these preferences quickly disappear as the professional asks relevant questions and makes reasonable suggestions. These questions and suggestions reveal you to be the calmest, most knowledgeable person in the room. In trying to help patients, no one, male or female, gay, straight, or trans, has ever asked me about my sexual life. If one of your patients does, you have several good response options. You can warmly smile and ask if you can learn why this is important to him or her; you can calmly say that you prefer to keep the focus of conversations on the patient or the couple; you can remind the man or the couple that all human beings, including therapists, experience concerns about their sexuality at times; you can remind the patient that ethical therapy requires a distinct boundary to prevent revelation about the doctor's personal life. Of course, you can combine elements of these four responses in your own creative way. Whatever you may say, your calm, warm, purposeful manner will sustain the alliance with the patient.

Two Extremes of Ejaculation

To further illuminate premature ejaculation, let us assume for the moment that intravaginal ejaculation times are distributed reasonably close to the classic bell-shaped curve of many other human characteristics. On the left side of the curve far from the mean we have men with premature ejaculation, with time to ejaculation of, say, 30 seconds or less. On the right side of the curve, far from the mean, we have men who have a difficult time ejaculating in the vagina—those with a time to ejaculation of 15 minutes or more, including those who cannot ejaculate in the vagina. It is likely that at either end of the spectrum of intravaginal times to ejaculation there exists an undiscovered specific biochemical or neural substrate that predisposes the men to their patterns. The problem is that science has not identified how this substrate differs from that in "normal" men. Very little understanding exists about the pathophysiology of delayed ejaculation.[14] Its biological substrate is unknown, and its medication treatment is largely a failure. I treat delayed ejaculation with psychotherapy, but it rarely improves quickly. It can resolve with psychotherapy. It is a different problem than premature ejaculation.

My clinical experience with both of these problematic ejaculation patterns returns me to the four bedrock forces that shape all of our sexualities. If we eventually discover that men with lifelong premature ejaculation have a genetic variation of the serotonin transporter in the upper cervical spinal cord or brain stem, a different gene sequence at one of the serotonin receptor sites (pathogenesis!),[15,16] or cerebral and thalamic white matter thickening,[17] they will continue to have to deal with their psychology, interpersonal relationship, and the clash between self-knowledge and cultural expectations for how a man ought to be sexually. The effectiveness of the medications does not obviate the need for a mental health professional. In fact, the mental health professional is needed for a much longer time for those with psychogenic delayed ejaculation.

References

1. Capsi A, Moffit TE: All for one and one for all: mental disorders in one dimension. Am J Psychiatry 175(9):831–844, 2018
2. Testosterone therapy for menopausal women. Drug Ther Bull 55(5):57–60, 2017
3. Koon CS, Sidi H, Kumar J, et al: The phosphodiasterase 5-inhibitors (PDE-5i) for erectile dysfunction (ED): a therapeutic challenge for psychiatrists. Curr Drug Targets 19(12):1366–1377, 2018
4. Wakefield JC: Diagnostic issues and controversies in DSM-5: return of the false positives problem. Annu Rev Clin Psychol 12:105–132, 2016
5. Masters WH, Johnson V: Human Sexual Inadequacy. Boston, MA, Little, Brown, 1970
6. Shindel AW, Vittinghoff E, Breyer BN: Erectile dysfunction and premature ejaculation in men who have sex with men. J Sex Med 9(2):576–584, 2012
7. Waldinger MD: The pathophysiology of lifelong premature ejaculation. Transl Androl Urol 5(4):424–433, 2016
8. Waldinger MD, McIntosh J, Schweizer DH: A five-nation survey to assess the distribution of intravaginal latency time among the general male population. J Sex Med 6(10):2888–2895, 2009
9. Verze P, Arcaniolo D, Palmieri A, et al: Premature ejaculation among Italian men: prevalence and clinical correlates from an observational, non-interventional, cross-sectional, epidemiological study (IPER). Sex Med 6(3):193–202, 2018
10. Choi JB, Kang SH, Lee DH, et al: Efficacy and safety of on-demand clomipramine for the treatment of premature ejaculation: a multicenter, randomized, double-blind, Phase III clinical trial. J Urol 201(1):147–152, 2019
11. Althof SE, McMahon CG, Waldinger MD, et al: An update of the Society of Sexual Medicine's guidelines for the diagnosis and treatment of premature ejaculation (PE). J Sex Med 2(2):60–90, 2014
12. Hamidi-Madani A, Motiee R, Mokhtari G, et al: The efficacy and safety of on-demand tramadol and paroxetine use in treatment of lifelong premature ejaculation: a randomized double-blind placebo-controlled clinical trial. J Reprod Infertil 19(1):10–15, 2018
13. Serefoglu EC, McMahon CG, Waldinger, MD, et al: An evidence-based unified definition of lifelong and acquired premature ejaculation: report of the second International Society for Sexual Medicine Ad Hoc Committee for the Definition of Premature Ejaculation. J Sex Med 11:1423–1441, 2014
14. Chen J: The pathophysiology of delayed ejaculation. Transl Androl Urol 5(4):549–562, 2016
15. Janssen PK, Schaik Rv, Olivier B, Waldinger MD: The 5-HT2C receptor gene Cys23Ser polymorphism influences the intravaginal ejaculation latency time in Dutch Caucasian men with lifelong premature ejaculation. Asian J Androl 16:607–610, 2014
16. Roaiah MF, Elkhayat YI, Rashed LA, et al: 5HT-1A receptor polymorphism effects ejaculatory function in Egyptian patients with lifelong premature ejaculation. Rev Int Androl Sep 25, 2018. pii: S1698-031X(18)30060-8 (Epub ahead of print)
17. Gao M, Yang X, Liu L, et al: Abnormal white matter microstructure in lifelong premature ejaculation patients identified by tract-based spatial statistical analysis. J Sex Med 15(9):1272–1279, 2018

3 | The Developmental Female Dysfunction

Varieties of Anorgasmia

The bodies of almost all girls, teenagers, and young adults are anatomically, neurologically, hormonally, and hemodynamically equipped to experience orgasm. The capacity for orgasm is a human characteristic whose absence requires some biological or psychological explanation. Many anorgasmic women ask their physicians if they are normal "down there," even though they menstruate regularly, have never previously had any pelvic or genito-urinary problems, and have no obvious relevant congenital abnormality. They may share that they have tried to masturbate with no success or never attempted this behavior, either because it was forbidden or because it had never occurred to them. They never, or almost never, have been able to attain what they think an orgasm is by any means with a partner. The professional will ask the woman if she feels sexual desire and can be highly aroused with her partner, trying to ascertain if the anorgasmia is the end product of another more basic sexual problem. She will respond affirmatively but often remarks that her arousal seems to suddenly fade away when she and her partner are trying to attain this goal. She recognizes from reading, pornography, or discussions with friends that the demarcating event is not occurring. However the professional may describe orgasm, the patient does not recognize having had the experience.

Orgasm consists of a sudden release of genital vascular engorgement accompanied by rhythmic pelvic muscle contractions and intense pleasure. The waves of genital pleasure seem to radiate outwardly to involve the entire body over 10–20 seconds. The woman is left with a sense of well-being, satisfaction, and ultimately a brief state of relaxation or fatigue as her genital structures return to their usual state. Many women eventually discover that they are capable of additional orgasms if the effective stimulation continues. In this way, orgasm is not followed by a refractory period as it is in the male.

Orgasm is also a more variable experience than in the male. Its intensity and duration may not be experienced in the same way from one woman to the next, or from one occurrence to the next. Its ease of attainment may vary from experience to experience. While the early studies of orgasm concluded that physiologically the bodily events of orgasm are the same regardless of how it is obtained,[1] subsequent magnetic resonance imaging studies demonstrate that numerous parts of the brain are involved, but not to the same extent and in the same location.[2,3] Some women report that their orgasms obtained in one mode generally are subjectively more intense than in another mode, which may or may not be the mode they prefer.

There are four important variations on anorgasmia. It is useful to know that although most of your clinical experiences will focus on patients in the first two categories, the third and fourth may apply.

1. Lifelong generalized anorgasmia in all sexual circumstances[*]
2. Lifelong situational anorgasmia with partners but orgasmic with masturbation
3. Lifelong situational anorgasmia with masturbation but orgasmic with partners
4. Lifelong unrecognized orgasm—orgasm occurring in a subtler, quieter form than the woman expects during either masturbation or partner sex

Since many of the women in the first two categories are able to overcome the pattern with assistance, it is important for us to have some concepts of why orgasm matters and how to enable these women to attain their goals.

---

[*]A college student had a two-episode sexual experience with a man she met while abroad. She was orgasmic with intercourse both times. In the years since, with or without alcohol, she remained anorgasmic. I consider her to be in this category. Never or almost never = all sexual circumstances.

The Importance of Orgasm

The ability to have orgasm with a chosen partner is a vital personal developmental accomplishment. It is additionally important because it is a relationship-building, relationship-sustaining developmental capacity. It provides the woman with a private personal confidence in her identity as a sexually competent person. It is a source of continuing motivation to engage in partner sex for most of the rest of her life, as it provides physiological and psychological rewards to her. It enables her to prevent her partner—male, female, or trans—from privately feeling inadequate as a provider of pleasure.

In the early phases of a relationship, an anorgasmic woman typically maintains her motivation to have sex with her partner. The stimulation that her partner provides is effective in creating arousal. She derives personal pleasure from the partner's pleasure in her body and in her very being. Lovemaking affirms her worth. But over time, as she witnesses her partner's regular intense moments of orgasm, she begins to have a decreased motivation to reengage. Of course, her partner's pleasure continues to be important to her, just less so. She wonders, "What is in it for me?"

Orgasm is not, of course, the central issue of her life. There are many other matters that compete for her attention. She may not initially be aware that her anorgasmia may be an undiscussed factor in a partner's decision not to continue with a relationship, but over time this worry arrives. Some anorgasmic women decide to fake orgasm so as not to disappoint their partners.[4] The prevalence of this problem ranges widely from country to country,[5,6] but in the United States it may be as high as 25% in some populations of physically healthy young women. Many women and men may think anorgasmia is a bit disappointing but relatively unimportant. Both partners may expect orgasmic capacity to appear as they accumulate more sexual experience together as she loses her inhibitions and trusts her partner more and as the partner relates to her body more skillfully. Many couples use alcohol or other substances to try to relax and become less inhibited. Some experiment with watching or reading pornography together before interacting. Sometimes, these strategies work. Pregnancy increases the vascularity of the pelvis, and some women discover in their second trimester that orgasm is attainable for the first time. But pregnancy soon creates an entirely new physiological and psychological set of challenges and distractions.

The consequences of untreated lifelong anorgasmia are worrisome. After a few years, the woman may lose interest in sex. "It's not really that important to me. I don't want to even think about it." Her sexual life evolves into a pattern of limited sexual interest and limited arousal, which can bring about new interpersonal problems. A couple's sexuality can devolve into the belief that it is the woman's duty or into a persistent attitude of "just get it over with." The patterns of anorgasmia and their consequences apply equally to heterosexual, lesbian, and bisexual women.

The Role of Masturbation

Masturbation, the rhythmic self-stimulation of the genitalia, begins in early childhood as a means of self-soothing. Many adult women report beginning to have orgasms in childhood by various means of self-stimulation and continuing to do so throughout life. Some recognize that their masturbation is a tool for regulation of their emotional states. Ideas about masturbation emanating from physicians have changed from the nineteenth-century view that it was evil, a source of illness that must be prevented.[7] In the early twentieth century it was declared a normal activity if not done too much (undefined, of course). By the 1960s, masturbation was understood to be a universal response to growth and development that is often encrusted with moral concerns. Enlightenment was the prescription. Today, cultural traditions, often but not exclusively religious ones, have made it difficult for some women to acknowledge their masturbation. This can make the initial presentation of the patient's history a bit uncertain when the patient reports that she never has masturbated. When I feel uncertain, I find a way to ask about touching of the genitals for curiosity or sensation without employing the term. Sometimes I learn that she has had the experience and felt great pleasure.

We assume that masturbation to orgasm acquaints the teenager with high levels of arousal and ultimately orgasm. Through these experiences that may occur over several steps, the aim is not just pleasure. It is to become calmly tolerant about the affective buildup of the genital pleasures that professionals like to describe as "genital tension."

Masturbation provides the adolescent the personal experience of her sexually aroused state, and gradually as she gets used to it, she explores different ways of augmenting her pleasure: nipple, vaginal, or anal stimulation. She is also getting to know her erotic self through her thoughts during masturbation. She comes to know her satisfaction with her gendered self, her orientation, and her intention (what she imagines being done to her or what she is doing to the fantasied partner). It is through masturbation that she comes to accept her sexual self and begins to look forward to her future forays into interpersonal sex. The trouble with solo sex is that it remains either undiscussed or prohibited in the family, and she thinks that it is prohibited as well in the community as a whole. In some communities, she is correct! Many girls still grow up with the idea that they will "burn in hell for this sin" or experience some related variation of its dire moral consequences. We must try to understand the teenager's grasp of how the world works when she confronts her masturbatory urges or learns that others perform this prohibited act. Peers may facilitate this developmental step by discussing their pleasures or reinforce the avoidance of these "bad girl" behaviors.

Do not get the idea that a girl must masturbate in order to regularly have orgasms with a partner. Some women who are easily orgasmic with partners have bypassed adolescent masturbation. It is just that helping a young woman to examine the idea that masturbation is a perfectly normal behavior that the majority of women privately have experienced often is a turning point in the woman's rethinking her relationship to her body, in learning about her genital parts without having to amalgamate them into "down there," and in conceiving a woman who masturbates to be morally and psychologically an acceptable human being.

> Mary initially sought help for anorgasmia. Quickly I hospitalized her because of her anxiety, depression, and suicidal and impulsive behaviors. I learned that she and her husband were having increasingly chaotic sexual relationships in their attempt to overcome her anorgasmia. They were engaging in activities that caused her intense pain. Clothespins on her nipples were the latest tactic. Such things seemed to affectively destabilize her after sex.
>
> Mary eventually became orgasmic in ordinary ways with her second husband years later. Before she remarried, she had the following illuminating experience. She had never masturbated, thinking that it was religiously forbidden. She was one of five best friends who still socialized 25 years after meeting in first grade. Upon my urging, she asked each of these women about masturbation. Each of their responses resembled: sure, those nuns did not know what they were talking about. This greatly distressed her: "What was wrong with me, that I believed that I would burn in hell forever?" She cried about this to her mother. Her mother, who attended Mass daily, explained to her that since Mary's father began dialysis, she had increased her own masturbation to comfort herself. Her mother thought this private act had helped her get through many difficult moments in her life even before her husband became sick. Mary used this shocking experience of her mother's frank revelation to reorganize her sexual attitudes.

Assisting the Woman Who Has Never or Almost Never Masturbated

Assisting the woman who has never or almost never masturbated is the easy part. We discuss her ideas about masturbation and where they come from. You expect to hear that her parents never mentioned the topic or had referred to masturbation as a sin. You inquire how and when she first learned about masturbation. What were her reactions? Did her curiosity lead to self-exploration? You ask about older sisters and their intimate talk. Do not be surprised to learn that an older sister's tales of sexual experiences and her arguments with their parents about her social behaviors solidified the patient's ambition to be a "good girl." Such questions are premised on the idea that the clinician holds more enlightened views on the topic—namely, that it is an advantage to learn about personal eroticism and sexual pleasures in this private manner and that most girls, in fact, stimulate themselves to orgasm at various intervals. We stress masturbation as emotional self-regulation because we understand sexual arousal to fundamentally be an affective experience that relaxes people.

Depending on your assessment of "who this person is" in terms of identifying information such as age, relationship status, physical health, religiosity, degree of sexual experience, and so forth, you may refer her to one or more of the abundant books, magazine articles, or YouTube videos on the subject, but more importantly, to another meeting with you. In the 1970s, when anorgasmic women who had not experienced masturbation were readily available, Barbach demonstrated that group therapy helped 100% of undergraduate and graduate students to attain orgasm through masturbation at home.[8] Strange as it may seem, decades later Dodson helped women attain orgasm in larger groups by teaching them, lying on mats naked from the waist down, to masturbate using their hands and vibrators.[9] The culture, led by numerous facets of feminism,[10] has normalized masturbation for girls and women; your patient has been left behind. One cannot help but privately wonder how this happened.

However you convey this in your own kind, supportive, patient manner, the chances are that you can help the patient to attain and permanently stabilize this developmental step of learning and to enjoy and use her body's capacity for her pleasure—when she sees fit and without enduring internalized moral opprobrium. The role of the mental health professional is to promote growth, to facilitate maturation. The capacity to self-stimulate to orgasm is a developmental step. The worrisome thing about developmental steps is that they are not permanently opened windows of opportunity. This is one of the reasons it is easier to be successful with younger women than with women over age 40. Nonetheless, even much older women sometimes discover how to use their bodies in this way for the first time. There are few absolutes in human sexuality.

Assisting Women to Become Orgasmic With Their Partners

Assisting women to become orgasmic with their partners is both more complicated and more nuanced than facilitating the previous developmental step.

This, too, qualifies as another sexual developmental task. We are able to convey several ideas that ultimately can prove to be helpful.

1. There are multiple ways orgasm in the presence of a partner can be attained. Some are the result of the woman's activity. Others are the result of the partner's activity. Yet others are hard to classify because the sense of the partner's arousal augments her arousal and triggers her orgasm.
2. Although masturbation has taught the woman that she can create her orgasm, she is at a loss to understand how she can create orgasm with a partner. In terms of intercourse position, this is most readily accomplished when she is not constrained by her partner's weight so that she can move her pelvis in a manner that maximizes the woman's arousal. For many women this is to be on top, to use the penis as an anchor, and to move her pelvis in a head-to-toe direction while her vulva is pressed against the partner's body. To do this, she has to believe two ideas: that the sole purpose of intercourse is not to please her partner and that it is normal to move her body vigorously for this purpose.
3. Creating an orgasm with her partner requires her to trust that her partner will not negatively react to her taking control of the movement during intercourse. She has to overcome her concept that her role is to adjust her movements to those that the partner dictates. She may have previously only conceived of intercourse as being thrust into as the source of her orgasm. This experience works for some women, but not for most. I like to tell her that she is in charge of attaining her orgasm. When I say this in front of her male or female partner, I almost always see an expression of relief.
4. The therapist does not dictate how orgasm should be attained; we only explain how many others obtain it efficiently. Commercial movies are misleading because the scenes are often brief and passionate, and the woman is often standing against a wall or sitting on a counter, moving up and down intensely on his penis, or on her back being thrust into, while she is loudly orgasmic. Most mortals have different recurrent experiences.
5. The passive means of attaining orgasm with a partner involves the woman being open to direct stimulation of her breasts, clitoris, vulva, vagina, and sometimes the perineum and anus, by hand, lip and tongue, or vibrator. In the passive mode, I suggest that she put her heels together because this invites easy access to her genital parts. This often leads to a confession that she keeps her legs close together. She may have many reasons in general, and specific reasons sometimes, not to provide such access. By manual and oral means, the partner is providing her with another example of her body as the source of her pleasure. The couple comes to learn relatively quickly what she prefers, and whether it is verbalized or learned

from observation only (many do not want to talk about the details), the couple reexplores these sensual opportunities over time in various states of her arousal. The therapist emphasizes access and concentrating on the sensations being experienced and allowing herself to do what her body tells her. The current therapeutic fashion is to discuss this as increasing mindfulness. We do not emphasize orgasmic attainment per se, because this is a product of her antecedent excitement, the partner's pleasure in her excitement, and her arousal in response to what she perceives both within and from him (or her).

6. Vibrators are used both for masturbation and for partner sex. Many couples, for instance, have intercourse from behind while the woman holds the vibrator on her external genitalia. The heterosexual couple takes turns having orgasms: he in the vagina; she, before or afterward, with a vibrator. Some couples use phallic replica toys, which may vibrate to create novel pelvic sensations. While many couples have come to integrate a toy into their lovemaking, some wish the vibrator were not a requirement for the woman's orgasm. Lesbian couples have similar means of attaining orgasm, including manually, orally, with vibrator, through humping, and by dildo stimulation. Some women occasionally employ a strap-on dildo, enabling partner penetration.

7. Most important to each of the ideas above, the woman has to trust her emotional safety with her partner. Specifically, she must believe that she will not be criticized for how she behaves, what she desires, or how she sounds; her body will not be the source of his or her distress, criticism, or fear; and her withdrawal of consent for any particular act will immediately be respected—nothing will be forced upon her.

Role of the Mental Health Professional

Some patients may hear or read about the ideas in this chapter but find the recommended steps difficult to attain because they are seemingly mysteriously tied to memories, both recalled and forgotten experiences. These are generally not pleasant memories. Many women have had far less than ideal relationships with their parents, siblings, and boy- or girlfriends. Some have had serious childhood illnesses. Others have lost a parent or witnessed their parents' destructive infidelities, virulent arguments, or violence. Some were taken sexual advantage of or experienced other forms of disregard for their youthful personhood. Other patients may not have such a difficult history but still need you to help them through these steps. These women are easier to help than those with more definably traumatic backgrounds.

The professional makes a suggestion. The patient acknowledges its reasonableness and intends to implement it. She discovers she is unable to do so.[11] Investigating her resistance to moving forward becomes the work of therapy. Why do you suppose you could not? What did it make you think about? Did you dream about it? Even when the woman has no immediate explanation, we listen to her conversation for the rest of session to see what may lay behind her inability to do what might be helpful. In a seemingly unrelated fashion, she may recall some painful earlier life experience.

While none of us can identify the sequences of healthy sexual development as girls pass through various stages to adulthood, stories of poor attachment processes, trauma experiences, and misfortune are likely to be interfering with the patient's ability to currently carry out the reasonable suggestions. We do not have to rush the process. Despite her past adversities, and despite her seemingly irrational fears about allowing herself intense sexual pleasures, she may over time be able, with our warm, supportive, calm, understanding relationship to her, or her and her partner, to use the suggestions and move on to the next psychological or interpersonal obstacle until she accepts that she is worthy of experiencing her body as the source of her pleasure. We help previously traumatized people to grow into normality, into sexual health. This is not a matter of a task accomplished in a defined number of sessions or with a specific technique.

Although therapists of both genders are capable of helping young women through these sexual developmental processes, most women find it more difficult to speak of their genital anatomy and sexual behaviors to male therapists than to female therapists. Most state a preference for a female therapist. In other cases, the treatment focus on anorgasmia with a male therapist may occur after the relationship with him has been helpful with anxiety, depression, alcohol abuse, and so forth. Trust has already been built, and referral to another therapist may be experienced by the patient as a rejection. Just as with a female therapist, all of the male therapist's comments and suggestions need to be focused on the patient. This is not a time for personal revelations of his experience with women. While she is working on the goal with her therapist, she may briefly experience images of making love with her therapist within her eroticism. While this should not surprise a male or female therapist, these fantasies are typically private. One does not have to ask, but if the patient volunteers, stay calm and ask if she can say more about what she imagined. Perhaps it occurs because you have already proven yourself trustworthy as a caring interested person. Sex, after all, is a nurturant process with a safe individual who will not demean her for her interests or arousal. I think of such fantasies as a step along the way to the goal. I encourage female therapists to think of these "homosexual" fantasies in a similar fashion.

The Partner Relationship

From a psychodynamic therapy viewpoint, we may assume that lying behind a patient's resistance to employing our suggestions is some important story from her past. When we bring this to the fore and discuss her associated affects and their meaning to her at the time of its occurrence, we hope that these repeated processes will enable her to separate the past from the present and to begin to experience orgasms with her partner. This sounds good in theory, but sometimes the therapist's concept is being thwarted by something in her relationship with her intimate partner that tells her it is unsafe. It is not that the therapist has been wrong about the influence of the past; it is that, in addition, the relationship does not seem caring to her. She continues to negatively appraise her partner.

Sometimes a couple will cancel a session because of an argument that seemed to have nothing to do with their sexual dynamics. Discourage such cancellations. We are prepared to learn about the nonsexual aspects of their lives. The idea that we only talk about sex and they must see another therapist to talk about other matters is ridiculous. We want to identify all the factors that are preventing the couple from a relationship that happily deepens over time. We may act like sex is a separate aspect of life from work, childrearing, physical health, emotional health, relationships with friends, and responsibilities to family members, but this is quite wrong. Sexual dysfunctions bring us to the processes of life, not just the sexual processes. The sexual processes of life are embedded in a developmental matrix consisting of nonsexual processes. They each shape the other. Sex is actually not a simple process even when it works well.

Some women's anorgasmia probably improves on its own as accumulating life experiences and maturation enable mastery of previous constraints. I have heard numerous times that a woman with long-standing anorgasmia learns to enjoy sex with her next partner or that she continued to think about what we discussed while she was in therapy and "finally it clicked for me." While we cannot exactly characterize what comes from her spontaneous maturation or from an infectious attitude of ease about sex emanating from the new partner's kindness, we are certainly glad to learn that what seemed impossible to attain in the past can occur in the future.

A bright, accomplished, gregarious professional woman married a man who was "perfect on paper." She had neither masturbated nor had any genital activity before marriage. "I was a good girl." After several children, she remained anorgasmic and had diminishing arousal during her dutiful sex. For years, her husband complained that she was dysfunctional, angrily calling her frigid and in need of psychiatric help. "Not us, not me, YOU!" She worried that he was correct because of her low self-esteem about her body and her dysfunction. "My breasts are too small, my nose is too big, and I come from a family when men are assumed to be wise and get the last word." She was dramatically unsure of herself despite her achievements, but it was also apparent that she no longer liked or respected her patriarchal husband. She was in an internal rebellion against the wisdom and authority that she had invested in her father, uncles, and brothers. Two years later, alienated and intent on divorce, she became readily orgasmic with a man she began to trust and love, a man so different from the husband who had been perfect on paper. "So, this is love!" Her personal sexual developmental accomplishment propelled her to further confidence in her ability to deal with the challenges of divorce.

References

1. Masters WH, Johnson V: Human Sexual Response. Boston, MA, Little, Brown, 1966
2. Komisaruk B, Beyer-Flores C, Whipple B: The Science of Orgasm. Baltimore, MD, Johns Hopkins University Press, 2006
3. Wise NJ, Frangos E, Komisaruk BR: Brain activity unique to orgasm in women: an fMRI analysis. J Sex Med 14(11):1380–1391, 2017
4. Cooper EB, Fenigstein A, Fauber RL: The Faking Orgasm Scale for Women: psychometric properties. Arch Sex Behav 43(3):423–435, 2014
5. Lo SS, Kok WM: Sexual behavior and symptoms among reproductive age Chinese women in Hong Kong. J Sex Med 11(7):1749–1756, 2014
6. Amidu N, Owiredu WK, Woode E, et al: Incidence of sexual dysfunction: a prospective survey in Ghanaian females. Reprod Biol Endocrinol Sept 1;8:106, 2010
7. Engelhardt HT: The disease of masturbation: values and the concept of disease. Bull Hist Med 48(2):234–248, 1974
8. Barbach L: For Yourself: The Fulfillment of Female Sexuality. New York, New American Library, 1975
9 Dodson B: Sex for One: The Joy of Self Loving. New York, Crown, 1987
10. Boston Women's Health Book Collective, Norsigian J: Our Bodies, Ourselves, Revised Edition. New York, Atria Books/Simon & Schuster, 2011
11. Donahue KM: Problems with orgasm, in Handbook of Clinical Sexuality for Mental Health Professionals, 3rd Edition. Edited by Levine SB, Risen CB, Althof SE. New York, Routledge, 2016, pp 60–70

4 | Introduction to Erectile Dysfunctions

I think of the penis as having urinary, sexual, and comfort functions. The third can be seen as many go to sleep holding their precious organ. Oh, the male genital has other uses as well. Grabbing one's crotch can insult another. Speaking about it can be a form of braggadocio or enticement. From early boyhood on, it seems to fascinate, please, and excite its possessors. On the surface, this chapter is about the capacity of the penis to become erect and stay erect during sexual stimulation. But, at a deeper level, it is about the disconnection between emotional self-awareness and the conduct of sex. This disconnection reflects a powerful internalized standard to be able to become and remain erect at every opportunity. The only relief comes from being old, but even those whom young people call old often react to their waning potency with silent embarrassment, shame, and anxiety. Younger men can be counted on to be quite distressed. This chapter is an introduction to the clinical basics. We have to incorporate these concepts before we can appreciate the complicated interpersonal dilemmas hidden under the complaint of impaired potency for many middle-age and older men.

Here are two stories to consider:

1. Anthropologist Margaret Mead asked a Polynesian elder what the word for *impotence* was in his language. "There is no term," he replied. Now extremely curious about this seemingly prosexual culture, she asked about whether a man ever lies with a woman but cannot maintain an erection? "Of course," he replied. If there is no word for this, she continued, how do you explain it? "He just might not have felt like it that night."

2. Five inebriated high school football team members were taking turns having vaginal intercourse with a barely conscious drunken classmate. The sixth boy in line could not become erect. His friends found his inadequacy humorous, but only later could he understand that his inability to become erect was preventing him from further participation in a morally despicable act.

The DSM-5 definition of erectile disorder requires distressing difficulty in at least 75% of opportunities and a 6-month duration.[1] These criteria are better suited for pharmaceutical research than for clinical practice, where we try to quickly respond to patients' concerns. Wouldn't you feel obligated to assist a recently married man who has failed to obtain or maintain a rigid erection on two of five occasions over the 2 months since his wedding and was "a nervous wreck" during the other three? I would not send him away with the idea that his condition does not yet qualify for a diagnosis.

DSM-5's term is rarely used. The problem we deal with is widely known as *erectile dysfunction*, or ED. ED has come to connote that something is amiss in the body rather than in the mind. Advertisements for phosphodiesterase-5 (PDE-5) inhibitor medications attempt to decrease embarrassment at seeking help for this prevalent problem in middle age. For many centuries, the problem was known as "impotence." In 1993, a National Institutes of Health conference adopted the term *erectile dysfunction* so as not to cast aspersions on the man's character and social roles and to emphasize the emerging conviction that the symptom was a result of pathophysiology.[2] These researchers were correct that these men do not like to be referred to as impotent. But some do not like the medical connotations of ED either. I refer to my patients' problems as having an "unreliable" or "undependable" penis. They clearly prefer these word pairings.

Three Major Conceptual Pathways to Erectile Dysfunction

A man's ability to become and stay erect with a partner rests upon his capacity to find the interpersonal sexual context arousing. His brain must have the capacity to transform his excitement into increased penile blood flow. This is done through neural impulses that pass through the spinal cord into autonomic nerves to the penile blood vessels in its two corpora cavernosal bodies and its one corpus spongiosum. These nerves run through the capsule of the prostate gland. Erection is the peripheral manifestation of the feeling of sexual excitement, just as tears are the peripheral manifestation of sadness. A man's inability to create or sustain this arousal during sexual behavior explains his flaccidity. The inability to sustain arousal is the essence of psychogenic ED. In organically caused ED, the man can sustain excitement but his body cannot transform his feeling state into penile blood flow. This condition can be seen after a prostatectomy for cancer. When discernible historical features of both organically caused and psychogenic ED are present, the man is said to have mixed ED.

Most of my patients have psychogenic ED or mixed ED. I have a bias toward identifying the personal, interpersonal, and cultural forces that generate unreliable erections. Urologists, who have been inundated with men with potency concerns since their specialty began in the mid-nineteenth century, see many more men with ED than do mental health professionals. Their bias is that most cases of ED not caused by a previous surgery or a medication are the consequence of a biochemical deficiency within the endothelial cells of the cavernosal sinusoids. They assume that the symptom is a harbinger of future coronary or cerebral artery disease.[3] Their literature rejects the organic versus psychogenic dichotomy and instead is active in investigating biological abnormalities and therapeutics. Urologists prefer to assert that ED is caused by multiple factors, with a preponderance of biological ones.[4] The modal age of their patients is about 57 years. Many have medical problems, particularly those that predispose to cardiovascular disease. Mental health professionals tend to see younger, physically healthier men, but all clinicians see males from adolescence to old age with these concerns. A turf battle between urologists and mental health professionals is not in the best interest of most patients. Mental health professionals have more time with each patient and a longer duration of professional-patient relationship. The advantage of urologists is their possible quick prescription of a PDE-5 inhibitor. When that does not work, they have numerous means of medicating, mechanically assisting, or surgically intervening to improve penile reliability. Perhaps half of my new patients with the chief complaint of ED had already seen a urologist or primary care physician and were not helped with a PDE-5 inhibitor medication.

Should You Routinely Send Your Patient for a Medical Evaluation?

Because the causes of organic and mixed ED can be vascular, neural, endocrine, intrapenile, systemic, iatrogenic, or the consequence of substance abuse and/or aging, it would seem logical to assume that a physician would be required to discern these factors. The general public, and many primary care physicians and mental health professionals, think ruling out organic causes should be the first step—that is, psychogenic ED is a diagnosis of exclusion.[5] However, because the causes of psychogenic ED are numerous—relationship alienation, guilt over one's behavior, infidelity, gender identity, orientation and paraphilia issues, depression, partner's anger at the man, the man's anger at the partner, anxiety about performance, and prior premature ejaculation or the inability to ejaculate—it would seem logical that a mental health professional would be required to sort through the possibilities.

When you are the first one to evaluate the patient, you can competently decide on the next step based on your understanding of his history. If a man can routinely obtain and maintain a lasting rigid erection under a circumstance other the interpersonal sexual context, his nerves, blood supply, and endocrine milieu are sufficient for potency. The histories of men with psychogenic ED demonstrate that at least one of the following circumstances is present: excellent masturbatory erections, dependable middle of the night and morning erections, rigid erections in prolonged foreplay, lasting erections with pornography, lasting erections when a specific fantasy is employed, potency with another partner (male or female), and erection if cross-dressed, wearing leather, or caressing feet. Often the patient himself recognizes that his problem is entirely psychological because he sometimes can have perfectly satisfying sexual intercourse and other times cannot. The benefit of seeing a physician is the reassurance that this is psychogenic. Beside the time and expense, the danger is that he will be given a PDE-5 inhibtor that will be expensive, lead to dependence on an unnecessary medication, or fail to assist him in the long run.

When the history of a patient with ED demonstrates that under most circumstances the penis only partially fills without lasting stand-up rigidity, we suspect there is a biological barrier to potency. We are particularly suspicious when the man says he feels aroused but his penis remains only partially erect and he cannot recall any exceptions for a long period of time. Performance anxiety does not mean the problem is psychogenic. It is the pattern of erection attainment in all circumstances that makes us look for evidence of cardiovascular disease, diabetic autonomic neuropathy, hypogonadism, opioid use, medication side effects (including opioid substitution therapies), previous cancer chemotherapy, pelvic radiation, trauma, surgery, or systemic illnesses emanating from disease in the lungs, liver, kidney, or heart. There is danger in not sending someone for a medical evaluation. Not only will psychological interventions fail to improve his sexual capacity; they may delay or preclude his opportunity to have his underlying medical conditions ameliorated.

Patients with indeterminate histories should be referred as well. Some cases are really difficult to discern if you do not attend to the pattern of erections.

An embarrassed college junior confessed to his physician-father that he could not have sex. The father sent his son to two specialists, who thought he had psychogenic ED because of his age and sexual inexperience. Two trials with two different PDE-5 inhibitors did not help. The drugs depressed him because he thought that he might need a drug for the rest of his life. His worried mother shared with me that unlike his two brothers, she never recalled seeing him with an erection when he was small. The patient reported that he, too, could not recall any circumstance in which he had a lasting, rigid stand-up erection. "I'm turned on with my girlfriend, but my penis is never hard enough to have intercourse." The same was true during masturbation, with or without pornography; with morning erections; and with his previous girlfriend in high school. "I'm a virgin, but I don't want to be." His potency was significantly improved but not completely normalized with a complex vascular surgery to correct a congenital penile artery defect.

ED may coexist with other sexual dysfunctional symptoms. When we determine that these symptoms predate the ED, we wonder if the ED is a consequence of the preexisting sexual difficulty.

A 35-year-old teacher sought help for several months of obvious psychogenic ED, which followed his wife's recently expressed frustration over her limited intercourse possibilities. Medication treatment of his lifelong premature ejaculation was quickly effective. My reassuring prediction that his potency would become reliable as soon as his premature ejaculation improved was correct.

There are cases that scream out for the mental health professional.

A slightly effeminate 29-year-old men's clothing salesman sat down and immediately told me, "I'm a sexual mess. Girls leave me after a month or so. Sometimes, I come immediately; sometimes I lose my erection. On the rare occasions I maintain my erection, I can't come. I'm so nervous about having sex that although I want to have it, I don't want to have it. It is easier to masturbate." When asked, "What do you think about when you masturbate?" the patient replied, "It's weird, but lately I think about a little girl being spanked by her father."

Erectile Dysfunction Acquired After Previous Adequate Function: The Most Common Form

When acquired forms of ED occur among married men, therapists turn their attention to what has been happening between the couple. We are prepared to hear about conflict, alienation, affairs, depression, substance abuse, troubles with children or stepchildren, financial reversals, tensions with in-laws and parents, and other challenges. When the ED arises immediately upon divorce, we want to learn about the ending of the marriage—the man's disappointment, sadness, guilt, and anger; his fears about a new relationship; how he is coping with his alone state; and how he is relating to his ex-wife and children. No author can accurately summarize all the factors that rise within the complexity of a failing or failed marriage, but I assure you that I have helped many a man regain his potency without the use of medication by discussing his internal conflicting feelings and his less than empathic responses to his partner.

> My former patient, now a 62-year-old recently divorced father of three children, a stably employed high-level executive, had spent a year with me in psychotherapy trying to save his marriage. His wife could not seem to end an affair that she denied continuing even in the face of convincing evidence to the contrary. He had always been able to have intercourse in his two marriages. His first wife died of cancer in her 30s. A bit overweight, he was taking no medications, and he had no other physical symptoms. He was unable to have intercourse with the two women he dated since the divorce was finalized 6 months ago. He was unable to become firmly erect despite each women's cooperative manual and oral stimulation. He was able to help each to attain her orgasm. "This is so ironic. With one of the women, I was rock hard sitting in the back of the movie theater necking through the last half hour of the film. Later in the bedroom, I was dead. Do you think this has to do with my divorce, doctor?" I smiled, "Of course. Let's talk about that."

Lifelong Erectile Dysfunction: The Most Difficult Form to Reverse

Most of the men with lifelong psychogenic ED are single, but occasionally you will encounter men in unconsummated or rarely consummated marriages. When there is an obvious impediment to courtship and marriage, the etiological diagnosis of ED is not the usual challenge; the therapy is.

> A rabbi referred a recently married 28-year-old scholarly rabbi whose previous arranged marriage, which had been unconsummated, ended in 6 weeks, after his wife experienced a temporary psychosis and returned to her parents. Ari studied for a living, occasionally taught Hebrew to children, and was financially supported by his parents and his community. His new marriage to a sweet, extremely shy 23-year-old woman was arranged. I quickly perceived Ari to be preoccupied with one idea at a time in an obsessive-compulsive manner. He was sloppy in his unvarying clothing style. He had touch sensitivities

and had avoided expressions of affection all of his life. He had had few peer interactions during his life; he never dated. He ignored his occasional erections, thinking that they would lead to sinful impulses to masturbate. This was not much of a struggle for him; he claimed never to have masturbated. His testosterone was normal. He explained that he was a bright person with Asperger's syndrome. He liked his new wife, also socially and sexually inexperienced, but he was uncertain what to do to make her happy in bed. She was eager for sex but dismayed by his preference to be touched on his navel, which made him giggle with glee; it did not create an erection. Over the course of 20 sessions, I instructed him in a basic way. He took notes; I had to repeat myself because he wanted to make sure he got it right. Slowly he came to enjoy seeing her naked, touching her breasts, stimulating her genitals to orgasm by hand, and putting his sometimes erect penis in her vagina. He began to report firm erections in the morning. He was never sure that he ejaculated in her, but he eventually could allow her to manually stimulate his penis to a muted form of orgasm. "Something white and sticky came out." He was very pleased with their occasional successes, but he had not ejaculated in her body. After a year of no communication with me, he called brimming with pride in his voice that his wife delivered a healthy baby a week ago. He declined a follow-up visit "for now." A year later, he called with similar news. Then 6 months later his wife called to ask if I would see her husband again. He never made an appointment.

You should expect to find a high incidence of mental disorders in your patients with lifelong ED. However unremarkable the presentation of men with lifelong erection problems appears to be, they should be directly asked about the three components of their sexual identity. Some of these men present with so-called sexual addictions. Others have drug addiction, alcoholism, obsessive-compulsive disorder, schizophrenia, or mood disorders.[6] Some are married to women who cannot tolerate vaginal penetration. Since most individuals with these same conditions are potent, these men require us to realize what is getting in their way. Many initially deny that which eventually occurs to the clinician, namely, they do not want to have sex.

The Anxious Beginner

Count yourself fortunate when you see an adolescent who seems to be mentally well but who has failed to remain erect on his first or first few opportunities. Although he has lifelong ED, the category should not be applied to him.[7] He requires you to normalize not really knowing what to expect, not really knowing how to do this lovemaking thing. It helps him to share his anxiety with his partner because she or he will likely admit to being a bit anxious as well. Typically I see these teenagers one to three times before receiving an "all is well" message.

Helpful Ideas

Although the following ideas can be explained at separate times to patients to good effect, they are actually four dimensions of the same thing. The failure to maintain arousal during sex has an important background. For men with lifelong ED, the problem has very little to do with the current partner per se. For men with recently acquired forms, the remote past is not as compelling an explanation as what has more recently been going on in his private life within his marriage or outside of it.

1. *The horse race.* Typically, the anticipation of, and actual intimate experience with, a partner is inherently exciting. For a penis to be unreliable in these circumstances, some other feeling must be present to compete with or eradicate the inherent excitement. We are going to call this feeling fear, but that may only be a front for underlying guilt, disgust, resentment, embarrassment, or jealousy. In some early experiences of intercourse, there is a two-horse race between Excitement and Fear, which is won by Excitement by a nose, with Fear neck and neck throughout most of the race. This useful metaphor illuminates why one can remain erect until intercourse is expected; why a man can be erect for fellatio but not intercourse; why 20 minutes of rigidity during foreplay vanishes when the partner suggests they move to the bedroom. The anticipation of entering the vagina so energizes Fear that it outpaces Excitement.

2. *A significant story from the past that is lurking.* The feelings that compete with arousal are the surface manifestation of memories, not yet distinctly recalled or not yet told to the therapist.

> When I met Tom, a successful high-level bank employee, he was unable to consummate his 12-year marriage to a woman who had been sexually abused as a child. It took him several years in therapy to reveal to me that his alcoholic mother twice tried to kill him after having intercourse with him when he was 12 years old. For Tom, marital intercourse was more like a five-horse race: Excitement, Guilt, Disgust, Anger, and Fear. Memories are rarely this dramatic, but they often involve sexual abuse, intensely problematic parental relationships, or repeated attachment disappointments among orphaned, neglected, or fostered children. Tom eventually had intercourse a few times with a PDE-5 inhibitor, but he soon stopped trying. His wife, who had her own extensive history of sexual abuse as a child, smiled and said, "Oh, well, you can't have everything." The couple remained affectionate, respectful, and supportive of each other without attempting sexual behavior as they grew old together.

3. *The recurrent construction of a new reality.* You will meet men who ease their fear of sexual interaction by recreating a fantasy during the experience.

They quickly become absorbed in a private mental scenario, which is the actual source of their arousal. The usual fantasy involves gender transition, homosexual behavior, or a fetish or some paraphilic theme. The origins of these fantasies are often not recognized by the man. They typically are constructed to change some deeply upsetting childhood experiences. To make matters more difficult to discern for the clinician, they sometimes seem to be stimulated by something seen or read in pornography that efficiently excites the man. Whether this is because it taps into and reverses some childhood upsetting process or is simply broadly exciting across the population may never get clarified in therapy.

> Lance, an alpha male in every conventional sense of the term but one, had never consummated his marriage. What excited him were surreptitious glances at women's covered perineums, which he went to extraordinary lengths to capture on film so he could masturbate while watching. During his rare attempts at lovemaking with his wife, whom he always praised both as beautiful looking and as a wonderful person, he imagined seeing other women in pantyhose as if he were on the ground looking up when they were walking over him. It took him a year in therapy before he was able to talk about the incestuous aspects of his immediate and extended family's lives and their interactions with him and his sister.

4. *Resistance to understanding the fantasy.* You can expect your patient will much prefer his arousing fantasy than to return to the painful situations that gave rise to it. Once I interpreted a young husband's need for foreplay with his wife in boxing shorts and his asking her to don boxing gloves for a pretend match. Although he jokingly said to me that I had ruined his fantasy, the understanding gained in therapy allowed him to share with his wife at home his childhood humiliation over his unwillingness to fight a bully as his demeaning father demanded. His emotional conversation created a closeness to her that enabled them to put away the gloves and simply kiss and caress. Most of the time, patients do not respond this quickly.

The distinction I am making between lifelong and acquired psychogenic ED is not absolute. There is overlap. Even though a man with acquired psychogenic ED may have functioned with a firm erection for years in a heterosexual relationship, he often was tentative and anxious, used alcohol or other street drugs, used a fantasy to reach orgasm or limited his sexual encounters to prostitutes, never engaged in foreplay, only desired fellatio, or only had infrequent partner sex. Such a man is classified as acquired ED only because he found ways to have Excitement win by a nose. His form of ED invites you to explore his life history as thoroughly as you would with someone in a Fear-winning horse race.

I have one additional warning: an organic factor may contribute to psychogenic ED. The ability to separate psychogenic from organic ED does not mean that men who can masturbate with full, lasting erections and then experience difficulty with a partner do not necessarily have an organic factor at work. Masturbation is the most anxiety-free way to have sex. The man fantasizes some scenario, perhaps based on memory, to efficiently attain orgasm. With a partner, the man has to accommodate to the partner's sexual capacities and style, sense the partner's current judgment of him, feel the influence about what is going on in their lives outside of sex, and conform to vague cultural expectation norms. The attenuation of arousal from these concerns may allow a subtle organic defect to have impact. A man taking 40 mg of paroxetine for depression reported new ED. He elected to continue taking the drug. Two months later, he still had the problem at home but reported that during a 3-day affair at a convention he was fine with another partner. Biological forces (depression and the selective serotonin reuptake inhibitor) interacted with interpersonal forces (a marriage with known frustrating limitations and sexual ennui) and psychological elements (a new exciting relationship) to change the horse race.

Prognosis

Since Hippocrates, physicians have recognized that the ability to foresee future consequences of current conditions in individual patients is fundamental to the intuitive art of the doctor. While today there is a strong aspiration to make prognosis a scientific process of risk prediction based on evidence,[8] there still is much scientific uncertainty about prognosis for sexual problems, including erectile problems. What follows is the result of accumulating clinical experience rather than rigorous follow-up studies. For what it is worth, I trust these ideas.

Men with lifelong ED have a poor prognosis because they have experienced intense and repeated traumas, of various kinds, related to their sense of self. As we work with them, we appreciate the opportunity we have with the less traumatized men who possess better coping capacities. A few of the acquired cases are easy because these men have a discrete new dilemma that they can discuss in depth over time, alone or with their partner. They have the required courage, skill, memory, and vocabulary. With our guidance, issues that are formidable to them—such as a demotion at work, anger at a wife for her resentful disappointment about his infertility, and the gradual loss of psychological intimacy as the couple's workloads increased—are relatively simple for us to address. These situations carry a good prognosis if we help these patients see the pathways to their new symptom. We convey hope that an improved understanding of each partner's subjective life will create psychological intimacy. Psychological intimacy between them is what enables them to make love without the horse Fear.[6] In individual and couples therapy, the mental health professional creates psychological intimacy within the sessions. I suspect that the ability to enable patients to recreate psychological intimacy at home is what actually restores potency.

> Michael, whose diabetic foot ulcer had not healed in a year, was discovered through a phone call from his 25-year-old daughter to be at a strip club during his workday. Greatly disappointed and alarmed, she informed her mother, who was also shocked, embarrassed, and dismayed. She angrily noted in their first meeting with me that they had never discussed their last 2 years without sex. She thought the lack of sexual activity had been due to diabetes, and she had not wanted to humiliate him. She reacted to his confession of his weekly 2-hour lunch breaks with alcohol by declaring him "psychologically sick." We spent four weekly sessions discussing the motivations for his secret activity, his otherwise faithful behavior, his wish to stay married to his wife, his fears of his illness, and her feelings about their marriage, particularly in recent years. After the fourth session without any specific instructions, the couple resumed mutually satisfying intercourse. We stopped meeting after 10 sessions because their sexual activity persisted between sessions. "I'm done with strip clubs!"

It was useful to me to learn during the first session that he was often erect at the strip club before and during lap dances, despite having diabetic complications.

The Range of Therapies for Erectile Dysfunction

PDE-5 Inhibitor Medications

It is important for all professionals to understand how the PDE-5 inhibitor drug class works. In the United States, four drugs have been approved for ED: sildenafil (Viagra), tadalafil (Cialis), vardenafil (Levitra), and avanafil (Stendra). Some are available in sublingual forms. Sildenafil, vardenafil, and avanafil are more similar to one another than to tadalafil in duration of effect. Men can anticipate 4 hours of efficacy with the first three and up to 36 hours with tadalafil. Tadalafil has the slowest onset (1–2 hours); avanafil may be a bit faster on an empty stomach (35 minutes). There are no recommended food restrictions for tadalafil, but fatty foods and alcohol tend to delay the onset of action of the other three drugs. Patient preference is the usual guidance for treatment.

During sexual stimulation, the brain creates an erection through the penile nerves, which induce the release of nitric oxide from the endothelial lining cells of the three cavernosal sinusoidal bodies. Nitric oxide immediately binds to an enzyme, guanylate cyclase, which creates cyclic guanosine monophosphate (cGMP), whose role is to relax the smooth muscle cells overlaying the endothelial cells. cGMP accomplishes this by lowering the calcium level in the smooth muscle cells.

The function of the naturally occurring enzyme PDE-5 is to degrade cGMP from its vasodilating function. The physiological target of the four PDE-5 inhibitor medications is the same—to stop the degradation of cGMP. The inhibition of phosphodiesterase maintains the vasodilation effect of cGMP. The PDE-5 inhibitors can be active only after cGMP is formed. Without arousal, there is no nitric oxide released. If there is no nitric oxide released, cGMP is not formed and there is no change in the flaccid penis. Patients need to understand that their drug does not cause an erection. It keeps blood that has already begun to accumulate in the penis there longer.

There are 11 distinct types of PDE enzymes dispersed in the heart, brain, liver, muscles, adrenal cortex, retina, intestine, ovaries, testes, spleen, bladder, urethra, and prostate. The enzymes differ in amino acid sequences and in their sensitivity to PDE-5 inhibitors. The side effects of these drugs depend on their impact on the 10 other isoenzymes of PDE. The usual side effects are the result of vasodilation of capillaries in various body organs: headache, facial flushing, nasal congestion, muscle aches, and dyspepsia. Higher doses produce more frequent side effects. Rare side effects include loss of vision or loss of hearing.[9]

PDE-5 inhibitor drugs are not prescribed when men are taking any form of nitroglycerin because of the possibility of a dangerous hypotension. This constitutes an absolute contraindication. The drugs are used cautiously to avoid priapism when medications metabolized by cytochrome P450 3A4 liver enzymes, such as ketoconazole (which is used to treat fungal infections) and antiviral drugs (which are used to prevent and treat HIV infections) are taken concomitantly.

Before a PDE-5 inhibitor is provided, most physicians check the patient's list of medications and recommend elimination or reduction of those that are known to diminish potency. They, of course, are attuned to whether any underlying systemic illness can be better treated. Eradicating subtle congestive heart failure can improve potency, for example. Physicians may use this opportunity to urge the patient to stop smoking, drink less, exercise more, lose weight, and take his medications more compliantly.

The PDE-5 inhibitor medications can help men with all three etiological forms of ED. Many men with psychogenic ED prefer a drug to talk therapy. However, many men with this diagnosis come for psychotherapy after a PDE-5 inhibitor has failed to help them. It can be quite a struggle to convince a man dependent on a PDE--5 inhibitor to cease taking it even though he still has an unreliable penis. Sildenafil, which as Viagra usually was prescribed in 50- or 100-mg doses, is now available in a 20-mg generic form, making staying on the drug economically easier. Performance anxiety can maintain such counterproductive behavior until the therapist can demonstrate through the patient's sensual experience that the patient's potency can be reliable. After the patient's own improved sensuality improves, he can begin to focus on his partner's sensual opportunities, which only serves to further solidify his gains.

Other Direct Therapies Prescribed by Urologists

Ideally therapies prescribed by urologists, outlined below, are provided to those with accurate organic and mixed ED diagnoses and those with psychogenic ED that has proved resistant to psychological therapies.

- Intracavernosal injections of alprostadil (Caverject, Edex)
- Urethral suppository of alprostadil (Muse)
- Semi-rigid surgically implanted penile prosthesis (various types)
- Inflatable surgically implanted penile prosthesis (various types)
- Vacuum pumps (various types)
- Sonic shock wave therapy of penis
- Stem cell injections
- Platelet-rich plasma injections

The latter three interventions are known as "reparative therapies," a euphemism that is strikingly optimistic; they are not scientifically proven and not U.S. Food and Drug Administration–approved and yet are being given to many patients. Perhaps they help some men, but there is at least a strong possibility of a placebo effect. In the trials that led to approval of sildenafil, approximately 25% of patients responded to placebo (vs. 82% to sildenafil).

Role of Therapeutic Alliance in Psychotherapies With Men With Erectile Dysfunction and Couples

A therapy team consists of you, the knowledgeable one about ED, and the man and his partner, the experts in their life experiences. Together, the team needs to identify the locus of the problem as interpersonal or individual. The most relevant history often does not occur until a deeper trust is built.[10] Even when patients are baffled about the cause of their ED, they may know the specific antecedent events or processes, but they may not be ready to reveal them. The couple may not want to share with you, for instance, that the man's ED began after the woman developed a close relationship to a co-worker and suggested again that she was sexually unfulfilled at home. We have to be patient. Of course, with more experience we sense past events faster and we can zero in more efficiently on relevant issues.

> It took Fred and Jennifer three sessions to tell me "the truth." The ED had begun only after Jennifer refused to any longer play dress-up with him in full-length slips so that he could pretend they were two old ladies. Without the slips, Fred could not sustain an erection.

One of the most compelling reasons to see a couple together is that the couple affectively reacts to our inquiries about their subjective responses to past events. They share more of their inner selves in the process in front of us. After the session, they may feel closer to each other than they have in a long time. The new psychological intimacy of therapy increases their sexual desire and their hopefulness. The renewed sense of connection diminishes the man's worry about performance. They may then have intercourse that night following their first session. One of the earliest pleasures of specializing in sexual problems as a young man was the astounding experience of "curing" somebody. How many times can a psychiatric professional make such a claim?

Mental health professionals will more often confront serious interpersonal dilemmas caused by chronic individual problems. Conjoint work quickly exposes the couple's painful interpersonal dilemmas. The team of three then comes to see more clearly the tasks of therapy. The focus of treatment, which was originally on ED, may change to some other specific issue—the partner's drinking, a teenager's borderline behaviors, pornography dependence, and so forth. We soon learn what is transpiring in the children's, parents', and couple's lives. Even in the face of this widening realization of their lives, it is important to mention ED in almost every session. The team is working together to deal more effectively with their reality. I like to offer the idea that lovemaking is a safe harbor, a place of relief from dealing nonstop with their painful dilemma. Each of these metaphors—port in the storm, oasis in the desert, safe harbor—conveys to a couple that they are coping together with adversity and need to replenish themselves for tomorrow. Potency can improve without finding a solution for their dilemma. We work by defining their dilemmas, helping each person's views to be known, and sharing our sense that life traps everyone in something.

Individual therapy is also a vital approach. Since many men cannot discuss their histories in front of their partners, the therapist must judge when to see a man alone—often the first visit—and when to see the couple together—when they are quite clear that there are no secrets. The man often states his preferences on the phone. Meeting alone allows the man to speak about such things as his disappointments with his partner, his contributions to their alienation, his shame over sexual abuse, uncertainties about whether to leave the partner, and his secrets from her. Insight may emerge to the team of two that his unreliable penis reflects nonsexual matters. We come to see his existential dilemmas, other symptoms, strengths, limitations, and ambitions. The therapy of ED is an exploration of the forces that have robbed him of the ability to be present emotionally and sensually during lovemaking. After a short while both the patient and the professional see that the patient's unreliable penis is merely attached to his conflicted self. The penis can again become a far more reliable appendage for sex and comfort once he understands and processes what undermined it in the first place.

References

1. American Psychiatric Association: Diagnostic and Statistical Manual of Mental Disorders, 5th Edition. Arlington, VA, American Psychiatric Association, 2013, pp. 426–429
2. NIH Consensus Conference: Impotence. NIH Consensus Developmental Panel on Impotence. JAMA 270(1):83–90, 1993
3. Nehra A, Jackson G, Minor M, et al: The Princeton III Consensus recommendations for the management of erectile dysfunction and cardiovascular disease. Mayo Clin Proc 87(8):766–780, 2012
4. Jannini EA, McCabe MP, Salonia A, et al: Organic vs psychogenic? The Manichean diagnosis in sexual mediicne. J Sex Med 9:1726–1733, 2010
5. Montorsi F, Adaikan G, Becher E, et al: Summary of the recommendations on sexual dysfunctions in men. J Sex Med 7(11):3572–3578, 2010
6. Levine SB: Barriers to Loving: A Clinician's Perspective. New York, Routledge, 2014, p 133
7. Polonsky D: The sexual challenges for adolescent boys and young men, in Handbook of Clinical Sexuality for Mental Health Professionals, 3rd Edition. Edited by Levine SB, Risen CB, Althof SE. New York, Routledge, 2016, pp 111–122
8. Fusar-Poli P, Hijazi Z, Stahl D, Steyerberg EW: The science of prognosis: a review. JAMA Psychiatry 75(12):1289–1297, 2018
9. Shindel AW: 2009 update on phosphodiesterase type 5 inhibitor therapy, Part 2: updates on optimal utilization for sexual concerns and rare toxicities in this class. J Sex Med 6(9):2352–2364, 2009
10. Horvath AO, Del Re AC, Flückiger C, et al: Alliance in individual psychotherapy. Psychotherapy (Chic) 48(1):9–16, 2011

5 | Women's Sexual Desire: Life Cycle Perspective

Sexual desire is a central organizing concept of clinical sexuality. No topic can be thoroughly discussed without invoking it. It is integrally related to psychological and biological development, adolescent and adult relationship formation and evolution, illness experience, menopause, and aging. Biological sex and culture are major influences as well. I am hard-pressed to identify any major aspect of private and public sexual life that is irrelevant to desire. Individuals in the arts, literature, psychology, business, education, law, religion, philosophy, medicine, the mental health professions, politics, and the pharmaceutical industry have their unique interests in desire's well-known vagaries. The role of sexual desire in the culture, however, is different than sexual desire in clinical settings, where men and women and their partners often complain of a paucity of it, or, less frequently, of an excess of it. Professionals have devoted themselves for over 40 years to finding therapies for these complaints. Underlying this work has been one question: What is sexual desire?[1,2,3,4] Terms used to invoke the concept of sexual desire—lust, libido, drive, horniness, passion, interest, urge, appetite, instinct, sexual motivation—do not answer the question of what exactly is sexual desire.

Whatever we might eventually agree on as the fundamental nature of this phenomenon and its role in our lives, it seems to be understood that biological sex shapes its manifestations. It is not clear to what extent this is because of hormones, anatomy, pregnancy, paternal and maternal roles, cultural expectations, or social repression. What is clear is that biological males as a group have more sexual desire throughout life than biological females as a group. For both sexes, sexual desire manifestations are strongest in youth and young adulthood and often disappear in advanced old age. Nonetheless, discrepancies of sexual desire among couples—that is, tensions over who should determine the occurrence of sexual behavior—are nearly universal beyond the early years of a relationship. Menopause is a defining landmark for a decline in sexual desire for the majority of, but not all, women. These differences are relevant as clinicians struggle to define what is normal and what is not, what can be changed and what cannot be changed.

Despite all the papers and books on the disorders of women's sexual desire, there is still considerable controversy about whether the diminution of sexual desire after marriage and children is to be expected. Or, is the paucity of erotic imagery, the absence of sexual initiation, and the absence of the urge to masturbate among busy mothers in stable relationships actually abnormal? Women still seek help for their loss of sexual interest, but the help offered varies from clinic to clinic and from professional to professional. We have to guard against the idea that a diagnosis invariably leads to a particular treatment for all. We have been educated to believe that at least one-third of premenopausal women have a deficiency of sexual desire. One study of menopausal women put the figure at 87%. You would think, then, that it would be easy to find subjects to enroll in research protocols for medication treatment, but it is not. Prevalence data need to be treated with caution because desire concerns are often accompanied by arousal difficulties and results from study to study range widely, perhaps because different methods of ascertainment are used.[5] Nonetheless, studies converge on the idea that desire problems are frequent.

For my female readers, the knowledge of your personal sexual desires, your awareness of their waxing and waning, your responsiveness to what you see and hear and how you interact with others, and your experience of evolving within an established relationship will guide your understanding of patients' complaints. For my male readers, whether it is from participating in a relationship, observing the culture, or watching the arrivals and departures of your own and your partner's sexual desires, wisdom in this arena rests heavily on your own life experiences. Patients intuitively know this about you. It is one of the reasons people in their late 40s and older are uneasy about having a 30-year-old for a therapist. Their apprehension is based on the fact that you may not have lived long enough to understand. When this happened to me ("Oh, you look so young, doctor!"), I would ask them to decide at the end of the hour whether I seem to be able to adequately understand their lives ("Fair enough."). Despite the fact that readers may never reveal their personal experiences with desire with colleagues, I assure you that you know more about desire than you may think.

A Theoretical Synthesis: Three Components of Sexual Desire

I think about sexual desire in either sex as an elegant by-product of three ultimately inseparable forces that shape our individual sexual selves. Sexual desire may only be the sum of the forces that lean us toward and restrain us from sexual expression. Desire is highly context specific; it involves both conscious and unconscious considerations. Regrettably, sexual desire is often discussed in writings as though it was only one present or absent thing.

The Biological Component

Words like *drive*, *libido*, *horniness*, *instinct*, and *urge* are used to capture the spontaneous manifestations of this mysterious neuroendocrine, youthfully active, phenomenon. The biological component has an unmistakable basis in anatomy and neuroendocrine physiology; it typically diminishes or is tamed and civilized by maturation. Maturation does not eradicate drive; it merely controls its behavioral expression. Its sexual drive manifestations can be clinically divided into ordinary, high, and low endowments. The biological substrate for sexual desire diminishes over the life cycle, with a notable diminution with menopause. When a 70-year-old complains that she is "horny all the time," we recognize that this is a distinctly unusual state. When an 18-year-old reports never having felt any sexual feelings, it too, is recognized as distinctly unusual state of development.

The Psychological Component

The psychological component can be thought of as motivation to masturbate and motivation to engage in partner sex. The latter is the most important concept for us clinically. It translates into the degree of willingness a person has to enter into sexual behavior with a particular partner at a moment in time. Motivation is influenced by many factors: emotional states such as joy or sorrow; interpersonal climate such as mutual affection, admiration, disagreement, or disrespect; duration of the relationship; the needs of the partner; the woman's felt need for closeness and reassurance; and contexts such as being on vacation, reuniting after being away from partner, or being inebriated. Negative forces influence those with ordinary and low biological endowments more than those with high endowments. Exposure to other people's sexual enjoyment, whether seen, heard, or read, stimulates motivation for masturbation or partner sex. When a 40-year-old who had no sexual desire for 5 years comments that since she was freed from her marriage, she sexually feels like a teenager again, we smile knowing that single individuals have a strong need to connect with others and that unhappily married ones often feel erotically dead in relationships with their mates.

The Cultural Component

Families, schools, religious institutions, political processes, country of origin influences, historical influences, and economic forces can shape a person's awareness of personal sexual desire. These influences begin in childhood and can change as individuals are exposed to new ideas and different cultures. The mind screens all personal sexual behaviors with two questions: Is the behavior abnormal? Is it morally unacceptable? The answer to the first question reflects an understanding of the world, while the answer to the second one reflects the person's conscience. Values augment or diminish sexual desire by affecting our willingness to engage in sexual behaviors.

Cultural forces are insidious. In the nineteenth century, when masturbation was viewed as a public health menace, in regions where the populace knew that the devil resided in the "flesh," or when women were expected to provide sexual pleasure but not experience it, the chances of growing up at ease with sexual expression were limited.[6] Today in the United States women are expected to have desire and experience sexual fulfillment.

> A 34-year-old former nun became concerned when she courted a kind man she would have liked to marry but for the fact that she felt so uneasy about and almost repulsed by his interest in lovemaking. She had spent most of her life avoiding sexual feelings.

Of Course Women Are Not All Alike

It is instructive to look at two models of women's desire and how well they fit women's own evaluation of their experiences. There is no reason for clinicians to pledge allegiance to these models. Each seems to capture some women's experience.[7,8] A linear model offers desire as the forerunner of behavior that provokes arousal through masturbation or partner sex. Desire, then arousal, then orgasm in that sequence. A circular model is far more nuanced. It offers that desire is not a requirement for arousal. Receptivity and incentive for sex may bring women to behave sexually without desire. Arousal occurs from foreplay or intercourse; then in its midst desire appears in her subjectivity. Women engage in solo or partner sex for a variety of reasons. Their felt desire may follow arousal or not appear, even though they enjoy the experience. In the circular model, desire sometimes refers to drive and sometimes refers to intensely wanting what is happening once arousal occurs. Drive and arousal are difficult to separate. Drive may only be spontaneous early arousal. The majority of women in studies did not endorse either model as capturing their experience, but a minority ascribed to each.[7,8]

It is instructive to note that DSM-IV had three distinct disorders related to desire and arousal: sexual aversion disorder, hypoactive sexual desire disorder, and female sexual arousal disorder. Because the distinctions among these disorders, particularly the latter two, were difficult for clinicians to make, the DSM-5 subcommittee collapsed them into one disorder, female sexual interest/arousal disorder. The term *desire* disappeared in the female portion of sexual dysfunction nosology.

In the past when I used to ask male patients if they had a satisfying orgasm with their partner on Sunday, the first of the month, what day or date would they want to have sex again, the vast majority of men would quickly specifically answer my question. When I asked the same question to women, the most common answer I received was, "It depends." When I asked, "On what?" I received a variety of answers. Very few answered "on Friday" or "on the 10th."

What are we to make of those like Abby who feel that something is wrong with them and request our services?

> Abby, a 37-year-old mother of three boys, ranging in age from 18 months to 6 years, worked three days a week because it was "better for me to have an outlet outside of the house." She reported that she and her faithful husband "almost always" agree on decisions. He was a good father, mild mannered and generally helpful, but did not always listen well. She ran two marathons a year and trained almost daily. She was active in the Parent Teacher Association, attended monthly book club meetings, and took her children to their numerous individual activities when she was not at work.
>
> The couple used to enjoy morning sex before their children were born, but after that one of the boys was always with them in their bed in the morning. Abby still masturbated twice a week to satisfy her own needs: "It is easier than trying to coordinate with him, and orgasms are more efficient." Abby would prefer to have sex with her husband; in practice, she had no desire to summon the energy required to have sex with him. When they did have sex, she was easily aroused to orgasm, but this did not create desire for future partnered sexual activities. Abby worried about what this might mean for her marriage: "He has reluctantly accepted the lack of sexual contact and has stopped bugging me about it, but I'm afraid that he might look elsewhere for sex." She characterized her lack of desire as "the one void in my busy, otherwise satisfying, life."

There are now two Food and Drug Administration–approved drugs for premenopausal women who are distressed over the diminution or paucity of personally recognized sexual desire manifestations. Flibanserin (Addyi) 100 mg is a pill to be taken at night for 2 months before concluding that it has no efficacy for the patient. Efficacy may appear as early as several weeks, however.

Flibanserin, an SSRI molecule, has a feared hypotensive interaction with alcohol, so patients are asked not to drink alcohol while taking the drug. This may be one of several factors to explain the lack of therapeutic excitement for this 2015-approved compound. The potential side effects of fatigue, hypotension, and nausea may be another and are the reason why the drug is administered at bedtime. Most mental health professionals with prescription privileges have little experience with the medication, which is probably most frequently prescribed in women's health practices. The newest drug, approved in 2019, is bremelanotide (Vyleesi), 1.75 mg in 0.3-mL suspension. This peptide is a melanocortin receptor agonist that is delivered subcutaneously in a single dose auto-injector. Like flibanserin, bremelanotide in pivotal trials improved subjects' experienced sexual desire and ratings of arousal and orgasm at a greater level than was reported in women treated with placebo injections. Nausea and temporary mild hypertension are the most frequent side effects, but a much smaller number of women noticed increased pigmentation on frequent dosing. The maximum use is one injection per 24 hours, but most women used four injections or fewer per month. There is no alcohol use restriction. As of this writing, bremelanotide is not yet available in pharmacies.

Abby's story raises a number of questions for clinicians. Do we provide these drugs in sequence if the first choice does not ameliorate her situation? Do we tell her that she does not have sexual interest/arousal disorder because she masturbates and can be aroused to orgasm efficiently with her husband? Do we tell her that she seems to be pushing herself too much and needs to pull back a bit on some of her energy-expending activities? When she was asked about this, she said it was her nature to keep busy. "I just think there is something wrong with me, but I'm not depressed. I'm a happy person! I have a good life." Do we think she is denying resentment toward her husband for not helping out as much as she thought he should around the house or not listening to her? When asked, she smiled, shrugged her shoulders, and said, "He's a man." Do we agree with her that her lack of interest in sex with her husband is a diagnosable problem, such as hypoactive sexual desire disorder or sexual interest/arousal disorder, or simply a motivational problem to be worked out? Drive is present; she seems to have no cultural prohibitions preventing expressing her sexuality with masturbation; yet, she cannot get herself to do what she says she wants to be able to do, ought to do—make love with her husband. She is motivated not to do so. Abby's desire exists in a paradox. She has a divided self in this regard. She is bearing a contradiction. Her predicament seems more understandable when we recall that sexual desire is the result of interacting forces of drive, diverse motivations, and cultural acquired oughts and ought nots. Sometimes we cannot make a clear DSM-5 diagnosis or know what to do to improve a patient's predicament. Welcome to clinical sexuality.

A Long List of Relevant Adversities

We try to separate acquired forms of women's complaints about desire from lifelong patterns. Sometimes we cannot confidently achieve this because past adversities may have dampened sexual ease and pleasure without stopping desire's occasional appearance. These histories frequently do not pose insurmountable challenges in terms of developing a hypothesis about the current and remote sources of inhibition. Very occasionally a woman will state that she has never had any desire manifestations in her life, raising the possibility that some genetic variation of the neuroendocrine substrate of desire is the cause. This is not far-fetched when you consider that genetic variations of single protein syntheses are known to interfere in various ways with reproduction. Why not think that the underlying neuroendocrine system that serves sexual function can be similarly undermined by genetic variation? When a person reports that she has never had much sexual desire, we are in no position to distinguish a genetic cause from a variation on a bell-shaped curve of normality. These may be the same thing. I can testify, however, that sometimes a woman with lifelong low sexual desire discovers in psychotherapy or in a new relationship that she had been suppressing her sexual impulses. Life experience frees her from her prior inhibitions.

For some women with cancer, the price of successful treatment with chemotherapeutic agents is the destruction of their biological generator of desire and arousal mechanisms. Detailed understanding of these mechanisms does not exist. Removing the ovaries without replacement therapy, including androgens, can create the same situation in younger women without cancer. Physicians are afraid to provide breast cancer patients with androgens fearing that they will be converted within the body to estrogen, which might accelerate a dormant metastasis. As breast cancer affects about one in eight women, many of whom are premenopausal, this represents a prevalent problem for both single and partnered women. This is not simply a body image problem from a missing breast or a lumpectomy and its scar. Chemotherapies can eradicate eroticism and responsive arousal. This is particular evident in menopausal women. Other diseases that distort appearance may directly wreak havoc on a woman's willingness to be seen, fearing her partner may be repulsed. Even if the partner never admits to it, the woman may know that that is how the partner feels. I do not mean to imply that body image concerns are not important sources of withdrawal from partnered sexual life. Such concerns are just one factor among those who have had surgery and their partners. Obesity may encourage women to turn their interest from sex. Many other lifelong and acquired anatomic features that women consider unattractive may make it appear that they have no interest in sex.

Depression has long been recognized as a source of the loss of sexual desire. Although there are important varieties of depression, in general most represent treatable conditions with drugs that dampen sexual desire and arousal. There is a strong suspicion that many fail to recover their prior sexual functional capacities after the depression has resolved and they are no longer taking their selective serotonin reuptake inhibitor or serotonin-norepinephrine reuptake inhibitor medications. While it is reasonable to be concerned that the problem is a medication effect, we need also to consider that the circumstances that provoked the depression in the woman in the first place may have rearranged her attitudes toward and her interest in sex.

> One patient recounted, "Shortly after I discovered that my husband was having a 2-year affair, I developed migraine headaches and then fell into a depression thinking that my world had fallen apart. I eventually got myself together with a little professional help and took sertraline and decided for a host of reasons to grant his wish to stay married. Life has returned to normal except that I don't want to have sex with him. I don't know how long this will last; it has already been almost 2 years. When I think of having sex, it would be to please him—he is a nice person—but then I see him with her in my mind and lose my inclination. I don't think I'm simply punishing him, although there is that element. I think he thinks my 'trauma' is over since we talked about it at some length in therapy. Just because I don't bring it up doesn't mean I'm over it."

Psychotic illnesses and bipolar disorder can produce sexual excesses and deficiencies. The effects of these conditions are more complex than merely creating changes in desire. They involve impaired social judgments emanating from distortions in the sense of reality. When acute, they are cared for by psychiatrists, but many other mental health professionals take care of these individuals before and after the acute phases.

Of course, sexual motivation, if not drive itself, is typically diminished when unresolvable nonsexual conflicts emerge to alienate partners from each other. This is relevant to mental health professionals because women in this situation may not realize the impact of their anger on their sexual disinterest, may deny the degree of alienation, or may never bring up the absence of sexual desire and sexual behavior in therapy for other problems. It is one of the reasons mental health professionals have an advantage over medical professionals when considering the pathways to the loss of desire. We hear about the situation over many sessions, and we witness the changes in feelings about the spouse from time to time. However, if we don't see the patient very often, we may sometimes be surprised by the seemingly sudden decision to divorce. Women and men may represent themselves as loving their spouse. Even in these situations, mental health professionals are privileged to hear about the ambivalence of that love. Medical professionals are focused on diagnostic criteria and tend to intervene on that basis if a medication is available. In a 20- to 30-minute visit with the gynecologist that includes a pelvic examination, a patient who expresses her concern about decreased desire is more likely to discuss a medication as the first step than had she visited a mental health professional.

Past childhood and adolescent adversities present more complex challenges for both acquired and lifelong forms of desire deficiencies. They can be discerned, labeled, and discussed at length, with particular focus on the affects experienced when they occurred. But this humane process does not necessarily induce the woman to trust, feel safe with her partner, and become motivated to regain her body as a source of pleasure. Various adversities can have permanent consequences. I presume that the greater number of adversities in childhood, the more difficult it is to be sexually functional. My evidence is only that it has been repeatedly demonstrated that the greater the number of childhood adversities, the greater the likelihood of some adult mental illness. This pattern is even more apparent among racial minorities, sexual minorities, and those who are less educated, unemployed, or poor.[9] There is strong evidence that childhood adversities lead to neurobiological changes as well as those that can be understood psychologically.[10]

> Danielle, a 24-year-old college graduate, sought my assistance for her disinterest in sex, her discovered strong aversion in two relationships, and her fear that this pattern will continue to cause her to lose boyfriends. A bright, enterprising woman, Danielle had started a transportation business when she saw how students needed rides from the university to their homes in different cities. She had lived with her aunt for 9 years before going away to college. Her only sibling, a younger brother, lived with another aunt. They had been removed from their mother's home when their mother, who had schizophrenia, poured boiling water into their bath. After a brief hospitalization, social service permanently ended the mother's parental rights. Danielle, her brother, and her aunts have maintained connections with each other, but not with the mother.

These sad facts alone may have provided me with an indelible memory of what adversities some children endure, but there was another feature that made Danielle unforgettable. This additional element got me thinking about sexual victimization, vulnerability, ethics, and the uncertainty of the contributions of various adverse factors. For several years in her late adolescence Danielle had functional bowel complaints. When home for the summer, she visited an internist, "a handsome young doctor" who told her she was only expressing stress through her colon and proceeded to caress her vulva on the examination table until she had an orgasm. Nothing was said. She went back twice more with abdominal complaints with the same ending. The third time, the doctor seemed sure that she returned only to have an orgasm. She shyly asked if he wanted to see her outside the office. He brusquely refused. "I thought he cared about me," she confessed.

Sexual aversion generally means that the patient dreads sex, reacts with physical symptoms in anticipation, panics, or feels disgust when caressed. My sense is that married women with aversion feel it unwise to state their disinterest because of the fear of the partner's rage or violence or because they cannot find the words to express their contempt for the partner. I think that the woman would rather have her partner think of her as mentally sick than risk revealing how the partner disgusts her. Aversion can be partner specific, and it can reflect traumatic memories. Sex becomes the trigger for the affects associated with the original trauma. It is clinically satisfying to experience the transition from aversion to no desire for sex by simply helping the woman to recognize the experiences that gave rise to the aversion and to acknowledge her helplessness. Danielle lost her aversion and even enjoyed some partner sex, but she never attained a trusting attitude toward the two men she dated while seeing me.

The numerous adversities that you will hear about raise three questions:

1. What does a girl need to experience in order to become an adult with normal sexual functioning?
2. How does adversity undermine the process?
3. What are the protective factors that enable a girl to escape a dysfunctional state?

Let's consider some of the recurring adversities you will likely encounter: loss of closeness to a nurturant parent; loss of a parent through illness, death, divorce, or imprisonment; relative abandonment by the stressed-out remaining parent; loss of a nurturant parent due to illness in another family member; neglect, physical abuse, and/or sexual abuse often associated with parental substance abuse or severe mental illness; witnessing of domestic violence; personal serious childhood illness; and academic and social failures during childhood. When these adversities occur, several factors—how long they last, who is there to rescue the child, what useful distractions the girl has, what talents she has—appear to be modifiers of outcomes. Everyone with the same adversity does not have the same outcome. "Of course, my life at home sucked, but I was on three sports teams where I excelled and made good friends, some of whom welcomed me into their homes. I spent as little time at home as possible and could not wait until I was able to move out. Thank goodness for my grandfather." Sexual development may have more to do with numerous personal, nonsexual, subtle developmental accomplishments than sexual experience per se. These nonsexual processes lay the framework for coming to grips with personal pleasure as a safe harbor from the storms of life. Whatever their ultimate pathways are, adversities seem to interfere with basic trust in any partner's ability to care about them and in their sense of safety during sexual intimacies.

While the discussion thus far in this section has focused on identifying the developmental background of women's limitations of experiencing and expressing sexual desire within their ongoing relationships, many of these same adversities occur in the lives of boys. I see no reason to think that these misfortunes do not negatively affect men's comfort with sexual expression as well. Whereas women's sexual desire problems are thought to be their most prevalent sexual concern, limited sexual desire in men, which is still labeled hypoactive sexual desire disorder, may result from the same set of forces. Gender organizes many things, including professional perceptions. The same subjective manifestations, such as limited interest in partner sexual expression, get classified differently. Women are now categorized as having sexual interest/arousal disorder, whereas men are more frequently interpreted as having erectile dysfunction. Beware of overlooking diminished or inhibited sexual drive and sexual motivation in men complaining of their unreliable penile functionality. Sexual desire is inherent in all human beings; so are its vagaries.

Menopause

At every stage in life, biological, psychological, and social changes are simultaneously occurring because change, often too subtle to be apparent, is inherent in living. Going from grade school to junior high and high school to work, from single on birth control to married on no contraceptive, from pregnancy to motherhood to lactation, and from health to acute or chronic illness, involves many factors. Scientists wanting to know if menopause per se, whether naturally, surgically, medically, or radiation-induced, negatively affects sexual lives have used various methods to answer the question. The answer seems to be yes for many or even most, but not all, women. Abrupt menopause induced by oophorectomy or chemotherapy in previously menstruating women dramatically diminishes sexual interest and orgasmic capacity. Natural menopause is preceded by a perimenopause when vaginal dryness and hot flushes and flashes often begin while periods are less regular. After 12 months of amenorrhea, middle-age women are said to be in menopause. Several co-occurring processes make attributing a decline in women's drive and motivation to have sex difficult—duration of cohabitation, relationship status (single vs. partnered), hormone therapy, education, physical health, mental health, and relationship satisfaction. But a series of population-based studies over many years from different countries has consistently found that this stage is associated with a decreased frequency of sexual intercourse, orgasm, vaginal lubrication, and enjoyment of sex and sometimes is associated with urinary symptoms and weight gain.[11] Because this is widely viewed as normal, menopausal women whose sexual desire has diminished appear to be less distressed about it. Menopausal status is a more powerful factor than age alone.

Some women do not experience a decline, particularly in sexual satisfaction, and perhaps up to 10% note an increase in sexual behaviors. Much of this is explained by a new relationship but occasionally by freedom from worry about pregnancy. Studying the effects of natural menopausal transitions in large numbers of women is complicated by the diversity of women's relationship status: those without a partner (never married; divorced; and widowed); those whose husbands present sexual or behavioral problems that limit sexual expression; those who, although happily situated in their relationships, have personally lost interest in sex; and those whose sex lives have improved because of a new partner, resolution of an intrafamilial difficulty, or a mutual resolve to improve their sexual relationship.[12]

Prior to the publication of findings from a randomized controlled trial by the Women's Health Initiative in 2002,[13] medicine's response to the negative effects of the decline of ovarian hormone secretions, particularly estradiol, was hormone replacement therapy (HRT). In fact, women on HRT generally had better sexual lives than those who did not.[14] The evidence for the failure of estradiol with or without progesterone to protect from cardiovascular disease and the increased incidence of breast cancer and stroke dramatically changed prescribing habits. Today, after the findings from the Women's Health Initiative's study have been more thoroughly analyzed, women on HRT take lower doses of estrogen for shorter periods of time. Estradiol replacement is now thought to be more dangerous for women in their 60s than for recently menopausal younger women.

Increasing years after menopause is associated with the increasing incidence of vulvovaginal problems, which cause dyspareunia and tend to end a women's intercourse life, if not her entire sexual life. While we mental health professionals need to be aware of these problems, they are primarily studied and treated by gynecologists with a variety of methods, including vaginal moisturizers, lubricants, and various hormone preparations, including DHEA suppositories. Epidemiological studies of menopausal present an array of factors that influence the sexual experiences of women at this phase of life, but clinicians are called on to consider the woman in front of them at the moment. What is contributing to her complaints and what can be done about them?

Mental health professionals see many women for diverse problems who are also experiencing the physiological effects of menopause. For us, the issue is not the treatment of the symptoms that the gynecologists are attempting to ameliorate; rather, it is their problematic children, relational concerns, or the presence of depression, anxiety, addiction, or physical illness. Sometimes menopausal women want to restart their sexual lives and want to talk about their past negative experiences with sex. Not all women, of course, enter the menopausal transition with a history of consistent sexual pleasure. Some come to save their marriages, others to free themselves of their past sexual traumatic or unpleasant experiences, and others because they want to talk about their life processes with you. Menopause or their advancing years are just part of living. They want assistance with improving the quality of their lives. This is less a matter of medication and more a matter of sharing the past and present in order to be more open to the future.

References

1. Levine SB: Reexploring the nature of sexual desire. J Sex Marital Ther 28(1):39–51, 2002
2. Levine SB: The nature of sexual desire: a clinician's perspective. Arch Sex Behav 32(3):279–286, 2003
3. Rowland DL, Tempel AR: The enigma of sexual desire, Part 2: theoretical, scientific, and medical perspectives. Current Sexual Health Reports 8(3), May 2016
4. Toates F: How Sexual Desire Works: The Enigmatic Urge. Cambridge, UK, Cambridge University Press, 2015
5. McCabe MP, Sharlip ID, Lewis R, et al: Incidence and prevalence of sexual dysfunction in women and men: a consensus statement from the Fourth International Consultation on Sexual Medicine 2015. J Sex Med 13(2):144–152, 2016
6. Engelhardt HT: The disease of masturbation: values and the concept of disease. J Hist Med 48(2):234–248, 1974
7. Nowosielski K, Wróbel B, Kowalczyk R: Women's endorsement of models of sexual response: correlates and predictors. Arch Sex Behav 45(2):291–302, 2016
8. Giraldi A, Kristensen E, Sand M: Response and rebuttal of "Endorsement of Models Describing Sexual Response [of] Men and Women with a Sexual Partner: An Online Survey in a Population Sample of Danish Adults Ages 20-65 Years." J Sex Med 12(9):1981-1982, 2015
9. Merrick MT, Ford DC, Ports KA, Guinn AS: Prevalence of adverse childhood experiences from the 2011–2014 Behavioral Risk Factor Surveillance System in 23 states. JAMA Pediatrics 172(11):1038–1044, 2018
10. Herzog JI, Schmahl C: Adverse childhood experiences and the consequences on neurobiological, psychosocial, and somatic conditions across the lifespan. Front Psychiatry Sept 4; 9:420, 2018
11. Dennerstein L: The sexual impact of menopause, in Handbook of Clinical Sexuality for Mental Health Professionals, 2nd Edition. Edited by Levine SB, Risen CB, Althof SE. New York, Routledge, 2010, pp 215–227
12. Kleinplatz PJ, Paradis N, Charest M, et al: From sexual desire discrepancies to desirable sex: creating the optimal connection. J Sex Marital Ther 44(5):438–449, 2018
13. Rossouw JE, Anderson GL, Prentice RL, et al; Writing Group for the Women's Health Initiative Investigators: Risks and benefits of estrogen plus progestin in healthy postmenopausal women: principal results from the Women's Health Initiative randomized controlled trial. JAMA 288(3):321–333, 2002

14. Dennerstein L, Guthrie JR, Hayes RD, et al: Sexual function, dysfunction, and sexual distress in a prospective, population-based sample of mid-aged, Australian-born women. J Sex Med 5(10):2291–2299, 2008

6 | Betrayals

This chapter is the beginning of the second half of the book. Having shared what I think is a foundation for understanding sex through the life cycle, I now turn to the greater complexities that you will encounter in some of your patients' lives. As the culture has become more sophisticated about sexuality since the early 1970s, a greater percentage of requests for assistance involve the issues that will be discussed in the next four chapters.

At one time or another most mental health professionals who specialize in sexual dysfunctions have been overheard asking colleagues where the easy cases have gone. When their 1970 book *Human Sexual Inadequacy*[1] was published, Masters and Johnson created a revolution in print standards that enabled words like *sex*, *intercourse*, *masturbation*, *orgasm*, and *fellatio* to be printed without euphemism. These new standards were demonstrated in countless lay magazine articles and books, which must have freed many people from some of their inhibitions. These changes were co-occurring in some sectors of young people whose partnered sexual activities were increasing. At the same time, many mental health professionals became interested in sex therapy and helped a number of people relatively quickly. Nonetheless, I was doubtful about "easy cases" from my earliest experiences because I did not often encounter them. New practitioners tend to have an intense belief in a theoretical framework within which to view problems, including the sexual dysfunctions. In the early 1970s many in the new field of sex therapy suggested that past adversities could be bypassed through fantasy, through immersion in sensate focus (a guided series of touch exercises prescribed by Masters and Johnson to facilitate the sensuous state), through better communication between the partners about their sexual wishes, and through better education about sex. The new sex therapy promised a short-term, couples-based, give-them-information-and-permission approach that was a distinct departure from the emphasis on long-term individual therapy that had previously existed.[2]

I have been helping new and seasoned therapists take care of individuals and couples with sexual problems now for many years. I often hear them remark how complicated everyone's cases seem to be. I find myself smiling to myself, knowing that I, too, once briefly thought easy cases existed. Today, I realize that my early belief was misinformed. Occasionally I am fortunate enough to restore or enable adequate sexual function with a one- to four-session intervention. The vast majority of my patients, however, bring me their troubled lives, of which their sexuality is but one aspect. I am able to help many of them, but not quickly. Looking back, I realize that I have long accepted the ordinary complexity of my patients' lives. As I get older, I think I am getting better at delivering efficient care. I believe this can be your experience as well. So, welcome again to sexuality—this time to its more complex forms.

Reactions to Betrayal and the Therapist's Role

In discussing betrayal, we will begin to understand one of the sources of sexual dysfunction and psychiatric diagnoses, such as depression (despair), anxiety (intimations of disaster), and addictions (destructive self-calming). These parenthetical terms help us to appreciate the human experience of betrayal with a little less distance than our diagnostic terms otherwise provide.

While the usual form of betrayal that comes to clinical attention is infidelity, there are numerous other ways that a person can be betrayed. Those who may betray us include friends, siblings, parents, colleagues, a boss, an insurance company, a physician, government, a politician, and, of course, a lover or spouse. Experiences of betrayal are long recalled. The reactions to perceiving that one has been betrayed are similar regardless of what is the betraying behavior. If we place marital infidelity in the center of a line, there are lesser and greater types of betrayal on either side. The major emphasis in this chapter is on sexual betrayal in marriage or in established committed unmarried relationships. But parental sexual abuse of a child, for example, is an egregious betrayal of the unwritten basic social contract between parent and children to facilitate their health and development. Society in general has much stronger negative reactions to this form of betrayal than to infidelity among adults.

Therapists' Moral Judgments

Using just these two forms of betrayal—sexual betrayal in marriage or other relationships and sexual abuse by a parent—can introduce us to the countertransference challenges of working with people who have been betrayed and those who have betrayed. It is far easier to state that therapists are expected to be interested in learning about the life experiences of their patients while maintaining a neutral nonjudgmental position than it is to actually attain such emotional neutrality when dealing with these situations. Clinicians' equanimity is often challenged by situations of betrayal, because we do make judgments about matters that feel immoral to us. These initial judgments can be contained in us if we recognize that we are professional students of these situations. Organized society, through our professional license and our culturally esteemed role, allows us to be curious about how and why betrayals occurred. We may inquire of the betrayer at some time how he or she dealt with the widespread moral censure of such behavior without indicating any personal censure through the tone of our voice. "How do you think about this?" It is one our important professional learning goals to illuminate the process of betrayal in a kind inquisitive fashion to help patients to understand the antecedents and consequences of their behaviors. The subjective experience of not indicating our personal disapproval decidedly becomes easier to manage with just a few clinical experiences. It is initially more difficult for those who feel that they too have been victimized by a parent, lover, or spouse's infidelity. Nonetheless, the goal can be achieved by allowing your memories to occur and to remind yourself that you and the patient are separate individuals in differing circumstances.

Being Betrayed

I want to now return to the experience of being betrayed. The discovery of betrayal evokes an array of intense affects, changes one's self-concept, and alters how one sees the world. To the betrayed, the betrayer has violated a contract that immediately ruins the person's capacity to trust the betrayer. It induces a sense of superiority in that the betrayer is now viewed as lacking in integrity and honesty and is no longer worthy (of me, the children, and my extended family, in the situation of marital infidelity). The betrayed person becomes obsessed with vulgar angry descriptions of the betrayer. These express the sense of being violated by a disloyal act of treachery. The experience robs the betrayed of self-confidence. "I'm such a fool!" reverberates in the mind of the betrayed as the person realizes that his or her previous assumption that such an act would not occur because he or she was highly valued was mistaken. Waves of distress consisting of anxiety, sadness, disappointment, anger, guilt, and uncertainty about the future acutely dominate the minds of the betrayed, which gives them a subjective sense that they are going crazy or "losing it." The despair leads to indecisiveness, insomnia, panic attacks, poor concentration for other life responsibilities, and somatic symptoms such as anorexia, headaches, muscle and joint pain, nausea, vomiting, or diarrhea. Interspersed with the affects of victimization is a need for retribution, the wish to personally or have fate punish the betrayer.

When you see a betrayed person soon after the discovery of betrayal, all this is quite dramatic. You can be quite helpful to the sexually betrayed adult by recognizing that his or her affective waves are the leading edge of the search to find answers to four questions.

1. What is the personal, private meaning of the betrayal to me?
2. What is the best way I can respond to it?
3. Will I be abandoned?
4. Why did this happen?

The answers vary from one betrayed person to the next. The therapist's role is to educate the sexually betrayed about their affects and the questions these feelings are attached to. This quickly removes the sense of being crazy and stimulates the growth of self-knowledge, confidence, personal efficacy, and an appreciation of the predicament the betrayer created for both of them. In the longer term, the therapist and the patient come to realize that the affects, early answers to the four questions, and the understanding of betrayal in the larger world all evolve. The therapist knows that the patient's emotional environment changes as the feelings come to be individually experienced, labeled, understood, and given new personal meanings.

Reactions to Betraying and the Therapist's Role

Betraying evokes an array of subtle affects, changes one's self-concept, and alters one's understanding of the world. What and whom the betrayer betrays may include a school honor code, a premarital intimate relationship, a religious vow, a promise to another including one to a parent or a child, confidentiality, and, of course, one's previous or current partner or spouse. Betrayal involves indirect deception or lying. When betrayal is viewed this way, a large proportion of people have engaged in one or more of these behaviors.

Much is going on in the sexual betrayer's mind. Sexual betrayal involves a mental process of temptation, conscious restraint, defense, continuing temptation, justification, decision, and rationalization. Generally, the betrayer does not easily discuss this process or the personal reasons for overcoming the expectation of monogamy. The affects experienced by the betrayer seem to be far easier to contain than those of the betrayed. They do not typically present in a dramatic fashion. More often, they do not even seem to be present, or at least they are not readily discussed.

The therapist can be helpful in clarifying the betrayer's affects and questions. Many spousal sexual betrayers say they feel guilty and quickly apologize for the mistake. The guilt is not that intense, and the apology is not the same as remorse. Remorse is evident personal suffering over what one has done. The betrayer can be anxious about how to handle the partner's reactions and about the new negative social relationships that have evolved, or are threatened to evolve, in the family. The betrayer seems more preoccupied with management issues than personal affects. The betrayer is considering a large number of questions:

- What is the best way to manage this new situation?
- What do I want the relationship outcome to be?
- What do I feel about my partner now that I see what the discovery has evoked?
- How do I think of myself, now that I see what I have induced?
- Why did I do this?
- Is the problem that I got caught or is it that I did it?
- What do I feel about the paramour or my extramarital behaviors?
- Should I tell the therapist about my reasons or say, "I don't know"?
- How much of my motives and past behaviors shall I tell my partner?
- When do I declare, "Enough talk about this already?"

The therapist's role with the spousal betrayer is not to condemn. It is to clarify these separate questions for the patient because they too seem to be mentally occurring simultaneously, making the affects associated with each of them difficult to discern. While betrayers may feel bewildered, they often greatly appreciate the relief we afford them through pointing out the specific question that they are currently grappling with. These questions, of course, change with time. Although it initially seems more important to help the betrayer understand what the partner is going through so as not to completely annihilate their future possibilities, we also want the betrayed person to grasp the subjective processes of the betrayer. While betrayer and betrayed share a new predicament, they experience it differently. Your strength as a therapist lies in your ability to articulate the feelings and ideas that each person experiences but cannot put into words.

When betrayers of children are identified, they are considered criminals. Mental health professionals rarely have a chance to discuss their motivations, conflicts, justifications, and previous crimes at length and in depth. Forensic psychiatrists and psychologists may delve into the subject when evaluating a person who has abused a child, in or outside the family. Their processes are generally short-lived, however, because of the need to complete a written evaluation. Some corrections mental health professionals run group therapy programs with sex offenders. These programs often attempt to help these inmates appreciate the impact on the victim; their own history of neglect, abuse, or violence; and coping devices to deal with unpleasant feelings and dangerous impulses. By and large, the level of inquiry is far more likely to be in depth with the betrayer of a spouse than of a child. Therapists have a far greater chance to help an adult who has been sexually abused earlier in life than to help those who betrayed the victim by taking advantage of him or her sexually.

Grief

Grief is the ordinary response to loss of a person through death, prolonged separation, or divorce. It also is the expected response to the loss of a cherished belief, such as "My partner is faithful" or "I am a faithful person." When a wife discovers that her husband has been unfaithful in the commercial world of massage parlors, prostitution, strip clubs, or chat lines or that her spouse has been sexually involved with relative strangers through bar experiences or the Internet, she experiences a mixture of rage and grief. The abrupt cessation of these activities does not result in an intense form of grief in the betrayer, however. It may only lead to regret that this outlet is no longer available. "It's time to cool it."

This is not the case when there has been a love affair. Grief can be quite intense, although contained, for many people when their love affair is discovered. This is understandable because a caring bond had been established. The lovers have had growing valued knowledge of each other. Such grief quickly becomes evident in individual sessions where it can be expressed and honored. It cannot be deeply explored in conjoint therapy; it is too much to ask of an aggrieved spouse to recurrently bear witness to it and have sympathy. The therapist, however, can inform the aggrieved spouse about this consequence. I try to stop the betrayed from setting unrealistic standards, such as never contacting the paramour again, because it tends to only set up a repeat betrayal as the lovers reach out surreptitiously to say goodbye or to not end the relationship. This is an example of helping the betrayed understand what the betrayer is experiencing.

So-Called Sexual Addiction

The businesses of commercial sex, which are widely tolerated socially, economically, and legally, are thriving. Their customers often normalize their participation in it even while those who do not participate think the industries are not morally or socially wholesome. Men rarely seek therapy because of distress over partaking of the services of these industries. We get to see these men when their discovered behaviors lead their wives or partners to refer them for treatment with the label of sexual addiction. Occasionally, we see a former alcoholic or drug addict in treatment for depression whose counselor has discovered that he is now a compulsive user of commercial sex. When a spouse or her therapist labels a man as a sex addict, it is more about his infidelity in the commercial world or the pickup world of sex with strangers than it is about frequency of sexual activities. When the same behaviors occur among single and divorced men, there is no partner to betray. A label of sexual addiction is generally not used unless the man's vocation is limited by his participation in the commercial sex world.

Sexual addiction exists in gay male communities, but its perception is tempered by the well-documented fact that gay men as a group have more sexual partners over a lifetime than straight men. It may be more difficult to discern when sexual behavior is compulsive, is risky, and interferes with other important aspects of life. Sexual addiction may appear differently in clinics designed to serve the LGBTQ community and in HIV clinics. In ordinary clinic settings, married men who have compulsive sex with men tend to be seen more often than men who identify as gay.

We distinguish impersonal or commercial sex from a love affair because the meanings, processes, and outcomes are quite different. All commercial sex can be viewed as infidelity, but affairs of the heart, although preoccupying, do not belong in the heterogeneous category of sexual addictions. The motivations for sexual behaviors within this latter category and the underlying values that they reflect can be quite different from one person to the next, for example:

1. They have given up on their aspirations to love after the loss of a partner through death or divorce.
2. They never could tolerate sex in the context of ordinary emotional closeness/attachment.
3. They were introduced to pornography at or before puberty and were so overwhelmed by sexual excitement that their preoccupations interfered with their opportunities to experience an emotionally honest courtship.
4. They possess value systems that view recreational sex as a private entitlement.
5. They have newly been seduced by the discovery of arousal stimulated by relationship-less sex that is far more exciting than their marital sex lives.
6. They have been pursuing a paraphilic pleasure without which sexual function within an established relationship is not possible.

While the term *love object* would not be appropriate for the partners of these men, I am intrigued when others admit to thinking about and feeling love during their sexual behaviors. Some pretend that love exists between the sex worker and themselves. "I know I am in sexual Disneyland, but I don't care; it makes the lap dance more fun. I just pretend she loves me." "She was kind, she was into it, and I think she really liked me. I want to see her again. Being with her was not anything like being with other hookers. She told me she would be happy if I called again!" Others, the profoundly socially isolated, seem even more desperate to find love in their acts. A 30-year-old exhibitionist stalker who privately masturbates wearing pantyhose imagines that his young teenage victim will love him after he shocks her with his erection. "Yes, I hope that she will come to love me. There is a chance, you know!" Even though one might say that his low IQ and periodic psychotic episodes create this fulfilling fantasy of being loved, I am not sure if he is just being more honest than some others.

In 2011, sexual addiction was relabeled as hypersexual disorder, diagnostic criteria were articulated, and the DSM-5 committees were asked to approve it as a mental disorder. It was not accepted, even though therapists were engaged with helping many men to overcome their problematic patterns. Making an illness of these patterns posed many challenges. The criteria did not seem to fit frequent sexual behaviors in some parts of gay communities. Not only do gay men have fewer permanent partners to complain about their extradyadic behaviors, their committed partners are far more often accepting of them.

The original concept of sexual addiction focused on married men, some of whom were having homosexual encounters. Some appeared to be closeted bisexuals who were responding to their recurrent attractions to sex with men; others were heterosexually identified men who had been sexually abused as children or adolescents by an older male.

Single heterosexuals may have very different motives for commercial sex than married men. Up to one-third of men seen for sexual addiction have a paraphilic diagnosis.[3] Paraphilic drivenness is often present from puberty or before, but some men lose self-control of this long-standing interest only later in life. While all published series of sexual addicts are more than 90% male, few people think that women are immune to losing control of their sexual behaviors.[4] Their hypersexuality may only involve sex with strangers met in bars or on the Internet and masturbation with or without pornography use. An occasional woman attends Sex Addicts Anonymous groups. Bringing women and gender-nonconforming individuals into the topic of sexual addiction seems to complicate it. Gender can organize clinical perceptions. There was a time when the word *promiscuity* was only applied to women. Even today, however, clinicians are not used to inquiring about frequent sex with diverse partners among women who are not substance abusers or do not have bipolar disorder. With them clinical attention tends to be focused on sobriety and maintenance of mood-stabilizing medications, not their sexual behavior.

Male Sexual Addiction as a Barrier to Loving

Patterns of infidelity impede loving in conspicuous ways. Before discovery by the partner occurs, the man's time, energy, and interest are elsewhere. The partner explains away his disinterest in marital sex, with or without his deceptive help. When confronted by his pornography use in the home, he may normalize it or become angry over the concern and blame it on the partner's sexual unavailability. His past blame of the partner, minimum sexual involvement, and emotional withdrawal all come into a new perspective upon discovery and produce rage, alienation, and the new appraisal of him as person. Her new sense of him makes it difficult for her to love and abide with him. While for many the discovery of a partner's involvement in commercial sex or other forms of extramarital sex precipitates the decision to end the relationship, for others it creates a decision to withdraw interest, caring, optimism, and sexual behavior. The partner concludes that he will not be the source of much pleasure in the future. Relationships then become loveless endurance tests. What mental health professionals often hear from spouses is, "He is sick; you take care of him. Call me to come in when he is better."

After the crisis seems to have resolved and some conversations with the man have taken place, if the couple now wants to reactivate their sexual life, a familiar pattern may emerge. When the wife is again receptive to having sex and may want to in order to have a more fulfilling life, the husband may not be. They display the iconic psychopathology of love, the love-lust split. They cannot integrate affection and sexual pleasure in the same person. These men emphatically state that they love their partners and desire to continue the relationship. They are now much more involved in the partner's and the children's lives, but their love does not include a sexual component. The couple may remain without consistent partner sex for the rest of their lives.

> Ben said that his 40 years of "ridiculous" behaviors began with the discovery of his father's porn collection of she-males. This induced an aroused fascination with males with well-developed breasts and erections at age 11. It became combined over the years with visits to strip clubs; interactions with prostitutes; penetration of, and by, and fellatio of, she-males; placement of ads for sexual adventures; and masturbation at work to porn. At age 22 Ben found pictures of his mother having sex with other men and learned that his parents were swingers.
>
> Individual, group, and couples therapy enabled Ben to recognize the triggers and the personal consequences of his extramarital behaviors. After 2 years of therapy, he was able to stop them and to deal more genuinely with his wife.

It was always apparent that Ben, who describes himself as a very strange heterosexual, wanted to make love with his wife but never could generate the motivation to do so, other than for reproduction. His pleadings of exhaustion, headaches, or argumentativeness were eventually acknowledged as avoidance tactics and then ended. He claimed that what he had done sexually had made him undeserving of sex with his wife. "I hate myself for what I have done. I am so ashamed." Her invitations for sex were rarely accepted because of his fear of an inability to maintain an erection. The couple credits therapy for much improvement in their lives. He talks more. "I know more about what I feel now." We thought the problem had been overcome after they had three mutually pleasurable orgasmic intercourse experiences in a month. The sexual avoidance returned within several months, as did his pornography and prostitute use, despite the fact that his wife became a paranoid vigilant monitor of his daily movements and expenditures. "I understand her vigilance. It is fine with me. It helps me." He occasionally bickers about it, which diminishes the likelihood of sex. "Ben, when you complain about this, I know you are up to something."

Ben frequently reaffirms his love for his wife and their children. She has come close to ending the marriage many times, but it is apparent to her that they both love each other deeply. "Sexually I am a basket case, but don't give up on me. I really want to get better. You know this comes from my crazy family." For a long time this was the focus of their lives. Then came her cancer, which put his peculiarity and their love in a new perspective. Ben has had occasional slips but is generally better. His wife was and continues to be the initiator of occasional sex, and he remains a frequent decliner.

Love Affairs

In the United States the dominant public or political position concerning marital infidelity is that it is wrong, destructive, and a personal moral failing.[5] There is no term for the person who is unfaithful that does not connote a negative social judgment—cheater, womanizer, adulterer, slut, tart, floozy, and so forth. Even the word *unfaithful* conveys a strong negativity. Because all mental health professionals begin their training with a disorders paradigm, we tend to assume that all infidelity is a symptom of individual or relationship psychopathology. The ideas of immorality and mental sickness converge. If mental health professionals are not careful, we can become the agent of public opinion and assume the man or woman before us must have some sort of mental illness. You and your patient will be far better off if you assume that the love affair you are hearing about began as a decision made after calculating the benefits and the dangers.[6] The mental pathology—manic state, alcoholic deterioration, narcissistic or sociopathic personality, for example—has more to do with the judgment used to make the calculation.

Working with patients dealing with aspects of infidelity is difficult in the beginning, particularly when we have known infidelity in our parents, siblings, spouses, or ourselves. This stimulates our affect-laden memories and may provoke unwise countertransference responses. This typically involves directing them as to what they should do, such as Don't have an affair! End the affair now! Your partner is scum—you must divorce! You should have an affair of your own! Your marriage is over! and so on. Our role is to be interested in the person's dilemmas, and clarify the options, to enable the discussion to focus on what the person is thinking and feeling about the present, past, and future. That is all.

Affairs may be undertaken to restructure life. Sometimes they happen without this intent but do so anyway. Love affairs have a wide variety of outcomes.[7] I suspect that most are not discovered. Certainly, most are not brought to a clinician's attention. An undiscovered affair may continue to satisfy both participants for a long period of time, occasionally until death. It may continue to satisfy both until one person's psychological or social circumstances create a sputtering end that is difficult for each person. Grief ensues. Regardless, the energy required by the affair typically creates changes within the marriage. Sex becomes less frequent and less satisfying, and the one having the affair, perhaps to justify it, may complain more about, or to, the unaware partner. These changes are often felt by the spouse but are misattributed to some other factor.

When a discovered affair is the cause for either partner's decision to divorce, a whole new drama ensues that may involve you. Marriage to the paramour does not inevitably follow divorce. The drama of discovered betrayal is sometimes complicated by a pregnancy; a bout of major depression or substance abuse in the spouse, paramour, or a child; or a suicide attempt or suicide in one of the spouses, the paramour, or a teenage child. Any of these complications change everyone's calculus and emotional reactions. Even without such drama, affairs overtly or subtly restructure of life and carry short- and long-term dangers. Nonetheless, they continue to happen.

Why? This is a reasonable question.[8] No one can provide you with an inclusive list of explanations, although case by case you will inevitably begin to assemble one of your own. My only thoughts for you to consider is that marriage after a time may bring discomforting awareness of the self, the partner, or the future. And many people do not believe in monogamy for themselves. You can take it from there.

Individual circumstances in love affairs are far too diverse to speak of in other than generalities. For details in a specific case, the therapist must enter into a trusting relationship with the patient so he or she can teach one about the perceptions and thinking that enabled the calculation of benefits to be worth the risks. No one is asserting that the calculations are correct, are morally justified, or will lead to an improved subjective life. But when affairs are seen as attempts to overcome the impediments to love that are inherent in the partner or the self, or in their interaction, the particular case details become far less important than the human aspiration to find comfort through love. I just want to share two fairly typical cases with you. I am sure you will encounter similar patterns. I never considered Richard or Beth to exemplify love affairs stemming from major psychopathology. We can deal with those later.

> Richard had been struggling with intensifying homosexual desire since his last child moved out of the house after college graduation. His previous homosexual behaviors had been two drunken episodes in college. Married to, by his report, an anorgasmic wife who never seemed to like sex, this scientist said he wanted my help because of his depression and anxiety. He wanted only to talk, no medication. What he wanted to discuss was his discovery of the Internet gay community and the opportunities this represented both when he traveled and when he remained in town. His explorations eventually led to homosexual behavior that delighted him within several brief relationships. His dysthymia and anxiety dissipated. He and his wife had had periodic joking conversations about his homosexual desire. "You know you stare too long at handsome men." She commented on the fact that he had become happier. He told her about his two recent homosexual relationships. She was distressed by these revelations and issued ultimatums that he knew he would not, or could not, follow. He reassured her that he was not interested in leaving the marriage or humiliating her at church by coming out as a gay man. He refused to give up his new expanding friendships, however.
>
> After 2 years of continuing marital stability with fewer sexual initiations by him with her, he met a man who seemed a candidate for life partner. Their love affair caused him to ask for a divorce, and he came out to his siblings, parents, and young adult children, and at church. He was in pain primarily because of his wife's sadness, anger, and loneliness. Church members were supportive of both of them. He became preoccupied with the need to live independently and to work out a schedule for him and his lover, who lived an hour's drive away, to share their lives. This proved difficult. Eventually Richard learned that his lover, who was several years older, had not come out to his family. The partner's need to maintain his independence unraveled their relationship. Richard was brokenhearted. He thought of returning to the marriage. His depression was alleviated by several more brief but intense romantic excursions. Six months later, he met a man whom he thought was "the one." After 3 weeks, the man withdrew and Richard's despair was so intense that he could not work for a week. He requested an antidepressant. Richard's new gay friends were empathic throughout his panicky devastation. They reminded him that he was new at this. Although Richard remained on the lookout for a life partner, he came to see that he had to become more independent. "I count my blessings. I am still part of my family. I have new friends. I am healthy. I even attended a nude social gathering! I had never heard of such a thing. It was quite nice. Life is not as sexual as I thought it would be. It is very affectionate, however. But I still want to love someone. I want a man to love me."

Here is another situation of infidelity.

Mark's calm, pleasant happy life changed into the pain of betrayal and the humiliation of failing as a husband in an instant. Mark had trusted Beth implicitly despite the fact that he perceived that they never fully clicked sexually. Beth, who had been taking a selective serotonin reuptake inhibitor since age 16 when she had anxiety and compulsions, never complained about their sexual life. They were devoted parents, had many friends, and had cordial relationships with their local families. Over a 6-month period, her athletic skills progressed rapidly under the guidance of an instructor, who also taught their son. The coach one day shocked her when he declared that he wanted to kiss her. During the preceding months, Beth had begun to think that her husband was preoccupied with his career and seemed distant from her. After her next lesson, she said, "Just this once." This led to sexual intercourse within 2 weeks. Beth was astounded at how exciting the new sexual behavior proved to be; it was much more compelling than her quieter, four to six times per month, regularly orgasmic sexual life with Mark. Until then he had been her only sexual partner. Guilt led her to end the relationship after 4 months, but she quickly resumed for another 7 months. The lovers had no interest in leaving their families, never said they loved each other, did not talk much in person, and did not complain to each other about their marriages. They communicated by texting, saw each other at lessons several times a week, and had intercourse weekly.

Mark noticed that Beth was spending a lot more time away from him in their home. After he dreamt that she was having an affair, he checked her cell phone records and confronted her. She immediately cried in grave, shameful embarrassment, promised to end the relationship, and said that she wanted to stay married. When directly asked, she claimed she did not love the coach. She apologized repeatedly. She thought that no one else knew about the relationship. The couple agreed to tell no one about this. The next day Mark visited the coach, who corroborated Beth's story, apologized, agreed not to contact her again, and pleaded with Mark not to tell his wife.

When I saw them together, Mark was the most distressed person in the room. He said he was devastated, could not sleep or eat, had anxiety all day long, and felt pressure in his chest. After a month of individual and conjoint sessions, Mark decided he would remain married. He emphasized that he clearly was, by far, the better man. He felt he understood as much as could be understood about what happened. He was convinced that "Beth truly loves me and was getting over her coach. She made a very big mistake in judgment to get involved." On the 11th day after discovery, Mark and Beth began to have sex again. It was accompanied by an intensity that never had been there before. (I refer to this as "reclaiming sex.")

In this first month of frequent sessions, I was consistently interested in each of their viewpoints, concerns, and wishes for the future. Mark remained uncommitted about how things would work out until Beth patiently answered all his questions and maintained a consistent concern about his recurring emotional breakdowns. Initially, he could not understand how she could love him and sleep with another man. "If you did not love him, how could you have had sex with him?" He could not grasp why she did not agree that it was a poor idea to continue to take their son for lessons from that coach. Beth deferred to Mark's insistence that a new coach be found. As life was settling back to normal, Mark expressed his concern that Beth seemed too ready to sweep the affair under the rug. She did not want him to mention it. I gave him an analogy to coping with cancer chemotherapy: both partners are suffering anxieties but choose to lighten each other's burden by not fully discussing their subjective experiences. Another calm week occurred complete with weekend lovemaking. Each was busy with their usual tasks. He said the cancer analogy helped him protect her from his deepest worries. Mark felt that Beth was putting 100% of herself into him and the children again. He worried the affair was a response to a problem that she felt in the relationship which in the future might cause trouble. He feared that the shadow of another person would now always be intoxicating to her.

Beth worried about the meaning of always having to initiate their sexual opportunities. Mark answered, "Yes, but once you do, everything flows normally, and we are both pleased." Beth quickly asked, "But why won't you initiate it?" He was afraid to tell her the answer, but privately he told me that Beth disliked sex during college and he never wanted to force it on her, so he waited for her to signal her interest. That evening Mark was very sad, had difficulty sleeping, and felt that Beth wanted sexual things from him that he could not provide. She blurted out that she only wants Mark to indicate that he really wants her sexually. They had a long talk. He awakened in the morning feeling better, but she was sad, worried, disappointed, and confused. "I thought we had made progress but last night you were as distressed as you were a while ago."

They went away together for her athletic event and had the best sex of their lives. After the competition, she tearfully told him how grateful she was for his support that weekend, as well as during the trying previous 6 weeks. Mark was pleased. They had marvelous sex again before they returned home.

Mark asked me in Beth's presence whether anyone ever gets over this. Does anyone ever trust his partner again? This was my opportunity for a soliloquy. I explained that the Chinese write the character for *crisis* by combining the characters for the words *danger* and *opportunity*. I had seen that they were in grave danger. I was there to help them work through the danger in order to create a better life of their choosing. I asserted that many people get over a spouse's affair, but that I did not want to mislead them into thinking that there was no possibility of future unhappiness. Why would anyone aspire to forget that an affair occurred? I told them that I often dramatically pointed to my patients, accusing them of being meaning makers. "Beth's affair has different meanings to each of you. We all should act as though we know that over time meanings change, behaviors are viewed from a different perspective, and that which is painful can sometimes eventually be discussed more lightly. I neither want to trivialize what had happened within your marriage nor do I want to regard this as the worst possible thing that can happen in life."

Beth never wavered about wanting to stay married. The possibility that Mark ultimately would choose to divorce terrified her. Although she said she could give up the relationship immediately, she longed to communicate with her ex-lover. I explained that grief inevitably would be present because they were involved for a year. I thought it was dangerous to pretend that grief was not going to occur. Mark reversed his firm position by telling Beth that she and the coach could talk in order to help Beth to end their relationship. Beth reported that they spoke briefly on the telephone and texted each other for 2 days thereafter and stopped. When specifically asked during the first month, Beth revealed that she missed her paramour. After 1 month, she reported that she was thinking about him far less and did not miss him during Mark's recent absence. She missed Mark!

Words did not come easily when Beth tried to explain why she engaged in the affair. She acknowledged that she had grown comfortable with sex over the course of her marriage and no longer found it to be dirty as she did in its early years. She nodded in agreement when I asked her if their pattern of marital sexual behavior left her somewhat bored. She was curious what it might be like to be sexually involved with another person. The excitement of this relationship was far greater than she had ever imagined—"I loved being pursued!" She had told herself that she would be disciplined and discreet, that one day the relationship would end of its own accord and Mark would never know. She was shocked to discover how easy it was for her to conduct the deception. She had always thought that she could never be the kind of person who would do such a thing. She was mortified that her husband found out and felt profoundly guilty about the pain she caused him. She was ashamed of herself. When the questions returned in individual and conjoint meetings about why the affair occurred, she changed the subject to her concerns about Mark's mental health. Beth told Mark that she was telling the whole truth, but it was apparent to me that she minimized the frequency of sexual contact with her paramour and she withheld from Mark much of the process of her missing her lover. It was clear to me that she did not want to discuss the feelings that she had about the coach or her grief in any other way than to indicate her progress in getting past them. She canceled two sessions that she had asked for in order to better understand her motives for the affair. They canceled their last conjoint meeting with the message that they were doing well and thanked me.

The Dark Triad

Beth is not alone in the discovery of how easy it can be to be deceitful when there is some valued outcome. When Beth spoke of "not being that kind of person," I smiled to myself. I have heard this so often. What kind of person has an affair? We want the answer to be, a chronically dishonest person who does not care about the spouse's feelings, who is self-centered about everything in life, a real lowlife. People who have affairs are not like those of us who are free of major character pathology. I do not think this is correct. However, we do see men and women betrayers who have major character pathology. In these circumstances, I am used to discovering that the affair is the least of the problem.

One of my patients arrived as a couple to discuss the husband's obvious, but denied, infidelity. It seemed clear to all of us that he was in pursuit of being a big man in town. He frequently found ways to be with local celebrities. She benefited from their extravagant lifestyle but was humiliated by his cagey dishonesties and her discovery of the identity of one of his "friends." Her suspicions proved correct, although she knew little of the actual extent of his extramarital experiences throughout their two decades of marriage. Over time, his infidelity was dwarfed in importance by her unearthing his participation in an elaborate scheme to support and hide his opioid dependence. Although he saw me individually for a time, this was unknown to me. Months later, it became known that he was embezzling from his business partner, which eventually led to a threat to have him arrested. This did not occur, but he lost his lucrative business, which threatened his family's financial future. Today, as his wife reflects on her life with him, the affair ("or affairs") means little to her. She has bigger worries. He seems to her to be a pathetic example of a failed human being, one from whom she cannot wait to free herself when their legal problems are resolved.

In the literature of infidelity this is called the *dark triad*, a combination of Machiavellian lying, narcissism or consistent self-centeredness, and well-hidden psychopathy, meaning involvement in many less-than-honest activities.[9] The spouses of those who can be described this way have their own language for these terms. They have borne the burden of their partners' dishonesty, self-centeredness, and criminality. When more of the person's nefarious activities become known, the infidelity, per se, becomes dwarfed in importance. Therapists see all sorts of variations on these three traits, including those without criminality. These patients enable us to appreciate what a small portion of a person's life we may know about at any given time.

In the acute dramatic phases of discovered infidelity, the clinical focus remains on the partners' feelings, conflicts, questions, and symptoms. Over time, however, many other aspects of their lives come to be discussed: children, vocations, finances, families of origin, psychiatric problems, and so forth. This is not necessarily a defense against continuing to discuss relevant aspects of the infidelity that slowly emerge. It is often just an illumination of the many facets of their lives. These discussions in therapy stimulate further private thought processes that enable them to plan for their future, whether it is together or apart. Spouses come to think of their partners over time more clearly in terms of their characters.

The dark triad also reminds me that one of the challenges to staying in love is the overcoming of narcissism.[10] Loving people are able to put their own needs second to their partners and children. My interest in sexual life as a young clinician eventually turned my attention to love. Sitting with men, women, couples, and paramours who were processing their own or their partners' extradyadic sex helped me to clarify my understanding of this topic. Love, although rarely discussed by professionals,[6] inevitably comes up in therapy when people are sharing the details of their intimate lives.

References

1. Masters WH, Johnson V: Human Sexual Inadequacy. Boston, MA, Little, Brown, 1970
2. Kaplan HS: The New Sex Therapy. New York, Brunner/Mazel, 1974
3. Kaplan MS, Krueger RB: Diagnosis, assessment, and treatment of hypersexuality. J Sex Res 47(2–3):181–198, 2010
4. Turner M: Female Sexual compulsivity: a new syndrome. Psychiatr Clin North Am 31:113–128, 2008
5. Smith T: Attitudes towards sexual permissiveness: trends, correlates, and behavioral connections, in Sexuality Across the Course of Life. Edited by Rossi A. Chicago, IL, University of Chicago Press, 1994, pp 63–98
6. Levine SB: Infidelity, in Barriers to Loving: A Clinician's Perspective. New York, Routledge, 2014, pp 82–95
7. Atkins DC, Marín RA, Lo TT, et al: Outcomes of couples with infidelity in a community-based sample of couple therapy J Fam Psychol 24(2):212–216, 2010
8. Synder DK: Treatment of clients coping with infidelity: an introduction. J Clin Psychol 61:1367–1370, 2005
9. Josephs L: The Dynamics of Infidelity: Applying Relationship Science to Clinical Practice. Washington, DC, American Psychological Association, 2018
10. Levine SB: Demystifying Love: Plain Talk for the Mental Health Professional. New York, Routledge, 2006

7 | The Gender Revolution

The sexually conventional world—in academic terms, the heteronormative community—has historically had a difficult time accepting and understanding sexual minorities. Moral condemnation, legal persecution, attributions of inferiority, and discrimination have been widespread in society, particularly among those who are not part of the creative arts. This state of society has forced the sexual minority communities underground, meaning their gathering places have been largely unknown to the heteronormative world and their identities in the workplace have been largely unrecognized. This hiddenness sometimes applied to their families of origin as well. The term *sexual minority communities* previously only referred to lesbian women and gay men but today includes individuals who identify as bisexual, transgender, intersex, queer, and asexual—LGBTIQA. While the legacy of outlawing, punishing, discriminating, marginalizing, demeaning, and occasionally murdering still exists, much social, political, and legal progress has been accomplished.

Most heteronormative therapists whom I have met do not want to be viewed as belonging to groups who advocate any form of oppression of LGBTIQA individuals. However, the legacy of the mental health professions is that until the mid-1970s, homosexuality was considered to be a mental illness. Since then, being lesbian or gay has officially been viewed as a normal variation in the development of orientation. The history of psychiatry about this and many other matters raises the question, "What actually determines what is called a disorder (or illness, condition, disease, problem, syndrome, pathology)?" I do not want mental illness to be construed as a purely social construction—that is, of a time, of a culture, or of an intuitive unverifiable assumption about what is natural. However, I am aware that sometimes this occurs. "Witches" were burned at the stake, after all. Nor do I want mental illness to be construed as a purely biological construction except when there is strong

evidence that the individual's social milieu does not shape its genesis or resolution. The tragedy of dementia comes to mind. Today, DSM and ICD committees decide what is a disorder, what criteria must be met in order to qualify
to be in their nosologies, and with what other "diseases" the condition will be
grouped.

Definable Aspects of Identity

Before we discuss the mosaic of sexual identity that all of us possess, I want
to remind you that all individuals have multifaceted identities. Our professions have largely ignored identity per se, in favor of making diagnoses, helping people with their issues, or tracing problems to their families of origin.
Excluding the three components of sexual identity, I can think of at least 21
aspects of identity. *Identity* is generally defined as the answer one provides
to the question, "Who am I?"

1. Biological sex
2. Racial
3. Religious
4. Ethnic
5. Economic
6. Personal aesthetics
7. Vocational
8. Sociability (shy, socially avoidant, outgoing, gregarious)
9. Political
10. Familial
11. Spousal (single, attached, married, divorced, widowed)
12. Monogamous (nonmonogamous)
13. Intelligence level
14. Cultural
15. Dietary
16. National
17. Regional
18. Illness bearer
19. Caretaker of illness within the family
20. Recreational
21. Sports affiliation

These 21 aspects of identity are not equally important, and some do not
become defined within a person's lifetime. Each one of these is a limited
statement of a larger complexity. For instance, personal aesthetics opens up

the door to body image, the impact of being beautiful, average, or unattractive in self-estimation and the estimation of others. Aesthetics shape courtship processes. Each of these 21 aspects of identity can be passionately held. For instance, the political self may generate much heat, while the political identity of others is defined as misguided. Each aspect of identity can be life enhancing ("I love my work. I continue to grow in it."). It can be life limiting ("This is a dead-end job. I am so bored."). Or it can be life destroying (e.g., a criminal career can put a person in prison and then punish him or her for the rest of life because of felony convictions). Likewise, economic status, from poor to wealthy, can propel individuals to entirely different sensibilities, values, and opportunities.

This list defines individuality. Our uniqueness derives from the intersection of our identity components at any given time. For instance, all transgender people are not alike; they differ on many of the items on the list just as all New York Giants fans are not alike except in their interest in this football team. Many aspects of personal identity—for example, trans status or being a Giants fan—create a sense of kinship with others who share the experience.

Besides biological sex, which is based on immutable chromosomal organization, each of the remaining 20 items on the list changes over time. Some may change quickly in response to an event, whereas others gradually evolve as we pass from stage to stage in the life cycle. Consider religious beliefs. A person might be religious at 13, agnostic at 18, atheistic at 23, and religious at 55. In other words, the degree of emotional energy placed on any item on the list may dramatically escalate or diminish. Becoming a wife may be a highly invested idea during courtship and engagement, only to lose its luster after marriage. I liken identity to a kaleidoscope. Seen and unseen maturational forces cause its elements to realign into new designs from time to time. Instead of little pieces of colored glass or plastic, the kaleidoscope consists of pieces of identity.

In clinical work, identity is actually more complicated than the list of 21 identity features suggests. Personal identity also involves our character traits— kind, cruel, aggressive, stingy, generous, orderly, slovenly, self-centered, humble, independent, dependent, compliant, argumentative, and so on. Not only may the 21 identity features change over time, but our character traits may also evolve. A person is a changeable being. Eulogies often emphasize the positive traits of the deceased, attempting to capture the person's social or psychological essence. The work of the mental health professional with some patients involves helping them to modify some of their apparently problematic traits. "Can I help you respond to your mother with more kindness and interest in her perspective?" It is difficult to know when to end the list of identity features. If we were to include character traits, the list would become unwieldy.

Identity is further complicated by two additional considerations. The first is that the answers to "Who am I?" and "What are my major characteristics?" may be different from how we want to be known. Social identity is captured by, "How do I want others to think of me?" or "What do I want my reputation to be?" Of course, we cannot entirely control what others think of us, but our reputations are vital. Others categorize us in various ways. When we hear that "she is exactly what she seems to be," we become aware that others are known to have a degree of falseness about their social presentations. Whether it is an apparent lie here or there or an unfelt demonstration of caring, we sometimes sense that a person is not being honest or is being deceptive. This is a very difficult thing for therapists, because we want to assume that our patients' narratives are essentially truthful and not designed to achieve a particular response.

The second complication to our concept of identity is that professionals categorize their patients in terms of diagnoses and character traits. We are generally careful not to overemphasize our experience of them as people lest we rupture the therapy alliance. We label others as ADHD, bipolar, borderline, demented, autistic, and so forth. We typically do not think of these as identity labels. Diagnoses are, however, attempts to capture some essence of their current selves. The drawback of diagnoses is that they tend to delay our understanding of their uniqueness as a person. Nonetheless, how we think of them is vital to their health. For example, let's look at number 18 on the list, illness bearer. A patient's self-management of personal illness depends on the ability to incorporate the disease label into his or her sense of self. "I am a diabetic." The 15-year-old with juvenile diabetes who cannot yet do this may have recurrent bouts of ketoacidosis if he cannot accept this new, unwelcome label. Patients generally like our appreciation of their uniqueness. In medicine, the diagnosis is the first and most important matter. The patient's individuality is important, but primarily so that the physician can select the right treatment for the diagnosis. If a patient has pneumococcal pneumonia and is not allergic to penicillin, the doctor will give her that drug regardless of her identity characteristics. In our work, the individual characteristics of the patient play a far more determinative role in treatment. I mention this because many professionals who take care of individuals with gender dysphoria think that the treatment should be similar to that for pneumococcal pneumonia rather than to the treatment of depression, in which much depends on the individual's traits, identity components, and circumstances. In mental health work, despite their relevance to individuality, identity considerations are often ignored except in a few circumstances. Gender identity is the great modern exception.

The Components of Sexual Identity

The number of aspects identity is increased to 24 by the inclusion of three sexual identity components.

22. *Gender identity* (based on the sense of self in terms of masculinity/femininity)
23. *Orientation* (based on the inclination to create romantic attachments to, and have arousing sex with, a class of gendered others)
24. *Intention* (based on what one wants to do to a partner and have done to him or her during sexual activity)

The erotic features of these three components typically appear in consciousness long before partner sexual behaviors reflect them. Children and young adolescents may not have the words to describe the mental aspects of these sexual identity components as they are developing. When they are a little older, however, they are often able to talk about their attractions, bodily sensations, fantasies, and behaviors that indicate that they are moving in the direction of conventional or unconventional gender identity, orientation, or intentions. Individuals like to say to therapists that their sexual identities are normal—meaning, for example, males feel sufficiently masculine, and heterosexual, and want to make love in a mutual exchange of pleasure with a partner without demeaning behaviors or the intervention of a fetish. When one looks closely at the "normal," it is apparent that there is a range of identifications with masculinity and femininity, degrees of interest in the same sex, and, most notably, levels of interest in paraphilic themes. Because of this, I like to suggest that every person has a somewhat unique sexual identity. Sexual identity is in actuality a mosaic made up of identity fragments of gender identity, orientation, and intention. These fragments show up once in a while in dreams, masturbation fantasies, and behaviors with partners. We are more varied in our sexual identity mosaics than we ever let others know. Eroticism is a private matter, but it too is a kaleidoscope. When the evolution of the 24 dimensions of individual identity are considered along with the modifications of our character traits that may occur over time, it is clear that each of our patients is quite different from all of our other patients, even those who share the same diagnosis.

Gender Incongruence

Transgender phenomena are a modern version of the human developmental struggle for definition of one's personal and social identities. Children, adolescents, and adults of all ages and both sexes are now defining themselves in ways that were in the past deeply hidden in privacy. The incidence of these newly declared identities is increasing, at least as can be seen from the number of individuals who are requesting psychological, hormonal, or surgical assistance.[1] This is particularly true among adolescents who previously demonstrated no conspicuous cross-gender interests to their parents, teachers, and peers before puberty. This phenomenon is currently referred to as "rapid onset of gender dysphoria." The prevalence among teenagers may approximate 1/130, which means that there is likely to be one or more teenagers in most American high schools whose private identity or whose social expressions of gender identity are trans. To a trans adolescent and family, the single most important aspect of identity is gender identity. It is as though the other 23 dimensions and the young person's character traits matter little. This focus may also apply to some of their professional caregivers.

Rapid Evolution of Vocabulary

Two terms are highly relevant to understanding gender incongruence: gender binary and gender variant. *Gender binary* refers to male versus female. In the early years when adults requested a sex change, they were within the binary concept of sex being either/or. They were referred to as being *transsexual*. The gender binary concept used to be referred to as *gender dimorphism* (i.e., having two forms). In recent years, *gender* has more firmly replaced the word *sex* as the world has come to appreciate that one's gender can be psychologically constructed to differ from what is typically expected of biological males or females.

People who have no incongruence between their bodily sex and their psychological gender are referred to as *cis gendered*. This term includes all those whose primary and secondary sex characteristics do not offend their masculine or feminine styles of being. Cis-gendered people demonstrate an enormous range of how they may express their maleness or femaleness. Masculinity and femininity are varied and changeable behavioral expressions and subjectivities. It is only the language of gender that has recently created the term *cis gender*. There is nothing too homogeneous about cis-gendered individuals.

With the growing recognition that gender may have numerous evolving forms of identity and social expression, the term *gender variant* began to be used. Here is an abbreviated list of how some gender-variant people socially define themselves: transgender, gender nonconforming, gender nonbinary, gender fluid, gender queer, gender questioning, gender bending, queer, omnigender, pangender, agender, bigender, two-spirit, gender expansive. No one in this field will be surprised if next year there are a few more terms. The changes come from the subculture of trans individuals, not from the professionals who serve them.

Stepping back from gender incongruence for a moment, I want to suggest a formula for you:

Actual gender identity diversity = those who have changed within the gender binary + the gender variant + cis gendered

This formula may be confusing because it includes cis-gendered individuals. I have written it this way to emphasize the wide variations in how femininity and masculinity are defined in the general population of cis individuals, be they heterosexual, homosexual, or bisexual. Of course, sociologically today, gender diversity seems only to signify those on the trans spectrum. But when one has an opportunity to learn about what is contained within some cis-gendered persons' sexual identities, the formula is more relevant to human psychology.

Self-labels within the gender-binary or gender-variant categories represent only the beginning of this identity. How these individuals' gender identities will evolve is not clear, although many of the hormonal and surgical treatments assume that, unlike other aspects of identity, these patients' identities will permanently remain as they are today. Cross-gendered identified children, adolescents, and adults have been known to return to living in the gender roles originally assigned to them at birth.[2,3]

Forces Contributing to the Rising Incidence of Gender Incongruence

In June 2015, a half century of legal work for gay rights culminated in the Supreme Court's ruling to support marriage equality and antidiscrimination policies. In the decade prior to this decision, legal advocacy included the rights of trans people under the heading of minority rights. So the Supreme Court's decision proved to be a further rising tide for trans rights.

The Internet has played an enormously important role in ending the isolation of trans individuals and creating new virtual relationships, communities, and instructions on how to relate to the medical profession. Almost all trans people are immersed in social media. Some have suggested that this may be creating peer contagion.[4]

Celebrity trans people influence the young. This includes pop stars whose appearances are often gender bending. They model personal successful defiance of heteronormative standards. Trans young people often feel they are part of the revolution. They sense that they are overthrowing the established order and creating a vital social experiment that can only positively help those who are coming after them. This gives their personal struggles a larger purpose. Media coverage has largely been supportive as many editorialists have emphasized the courage required to present one's true sense of self.

Gender experts, with the credentials of the official policies of the American Psychiatric Association, the American Psychological Association, and the American Academy of Pediatrics, have declared that there is nothing pathological about alternative expression of gender.[5] They stress that social, hormonal, and surgical transitions improve the distress of gender incongruence and that the associated psychiatric problems are due to minority stress, which is both an internal psychological dilemma and the result of the external force of discrimination. They remind readers that making a psychopathology of gender incongruence is reminiscent of how the mental health professions viewed homosexuality prior to 1973.

These ideas have been met with a paucity of dissenting professional opinion, not because there is no disagreement,[6,7] but because transition-supportive treatments for trans patients are thought to be a sexual minority professional issue, and because some prominent mental health professionals have been socially, vocationally, and politically attacked for their views by trans activists.[8,9] If a young professional asks the reasonable question, "Are trans phenomena a sign of mental illness?" the answer may be given in sociopolitical, scientific, or philosophical terms. The safest and most succinct answer may be "Sometimes."

Diagnostic Criteria for Adolescents and Adults With the DSM-5 Diagnosis of Gender Dysphoria

DSM-5 defines gender dysphoria as a marked incongruence between one's experienced/expressed gender and assigned gender, of at least 6 months' duration, as manifested by two of the following[10]:

a. A marked incongruence between one's experienced/expressed gender and primary and/or secondary sex characteristics
b. A strong desire to be rid of one's primary and/or secondary sex characteristics because of a marked incongruence with one's experienced/expressed gender
c. A strong desire for the primary and/or secondary sex characteristics of the other gender
d. A strong desire to be of the other gender (or some alternative gender different from one's assigned gender)
e. A strong desire to be treated as the other gender (or some alternative gender different from one's assigned gender)
f. A strong conviction that one has the typical feelings and reactions of the other gender (or some alternative gender different from one's assigned gender)

In addition, the condition must be associated with clinically significant distress or impairment in social, occupational, or other important areas of functioning.

In actual practice the patient tells the therapist that he or she is trans. It is rare to meet such a person of any age in whom at least two of the six criteria are not met. More important, however, is the fact that now almost a third of the gender-variant older adolescents and young adults have not sought psychiatric evaluation, hormonal assistance, or surgical transformation.[11] These are gender-variant individuals, however they further self-define, who do not claim distress or describe impairments in social functioning. In middle and higher economic groups, they generally exist in undergraduate and graduate schools. Thus, we can diagnostically assert that people may identify as trans without the DSM-5 diagnostic criteria for gender dysphoria being met.

Differential Diagnosis

The medical concept of differential diagnosis refers to what else should be considered when making a diagnosis within the DSM-5 category of gender dysphoria. If the problem resembles gender dysphoria, what else might it be? The answer generally includes body dysmorphic disorder, dissociative identity disorder, paraphilic disorders, autism spectrum disorder, substance-induced or psychosis-induced, factitious disorder, and intersex conditions.

It is quite rare to find a person who says he, she, they, or zir is a trans person whose narrative does not fulfill the required 6 months' duration and distress criteria. Elements of some of these eight other diagnoses may be present in the person's histories. Patients may say that they hate their genitals, breasts, and/or facial or other features that mark them as a member of their repudiated sex. They may report that they cannot look at them. They may have a sexual trauma history that suggests a motive to avoid the helplessness that they associate with their assigned gender. They may find a parent to be reprehensible and may occasionally demonstrate signs of dissociation. Others may have traumatized them by bullying or violence based on their gender expressions, before or after transition. They may have been erotically excited by imagining themselves in a different body or by the clothing of the opposite sex before they consolidated their new identity. An underlying uncertainty about their gendered self may have led to substance abuse or psychosis. Or substance abuse or psychosis may have crystallized their new gender identities. Prior to declaring themselves trans, they may have been gripped with a restrictive eating disorder. They may have several hallmark features of autism.[12] Children in foster care have a higher prevalence of gender nonconformity than those in intact families.[13] In United States prisons, where there is likely to be the highest prevalence of gender dysphoria in the world,[14] one occasionally learns about inmates who are trans until they are released. When one learns of the intersex status of a person with gender dysphoria, it is useful to read about this esoteric state.[15]

Patients with gender dysphoria have more medical problems as they get older. It has long been recognized that there is a high prevalence of HIV infection among lower socioeconomic trans women.[16] This is often related to their work as prostitutes. Medical conditions that occur at an increased incidence in middle-age and older transgender populations include cardiovascular disease, cancer, asthma, chronic obstructive lung disease, and various significant infections.[17] These illnesses, along with suicide, account for the shorter life span (among those who have had sex reassignment surgery).[18]

Roles for the Mental Health Professional

In today's fast-paced processing of patients in clinics devoted to trans health, a vital developmental question is not considered: "What has led this person to repudiate the originally assigned gender?" Instead, it seems that the mental health professional is marginalized and exists to assure others that the person is not acutely mentally ill and does not have another, well-established mental disorder from the differential diagnosis list that needs to be treated first. The professional is then asked to write a letter to a hormone provider or surgeon recommending a transitional process. In this way, the ethical concerns of the subsequent physicians are somewhat assuaged.

I have a much more conservative view of the proper ethical role of the mental health professional than has been promulgated by WPATH (World Professional Association for Transgender Health) in its Standards of Care and subsequent institutionally derived-statements.[1] The assessment requires more time and is ideally accomplished in what might be called an extended evaluation, psychotherapy, or counseling. A thorough mental health evaluation rests upon a knowledgeable and caring relationship to the patient. I agree with institutional pronouncements (e.g., American Psychiatric Association's Task Force on Treatment of Gender Identity Disorder[19]) that psychiatric comorbidities such as depression, anxiety, suicidality, substance abuse, and autism, which are often associated with the diagnosis, should be carefully assessed. But my conservatism adds two other responsibilities to our work. I ask the patient:

1. Can we develop a hypothesis together as to why you are now repudiating your original gender sense?
2. Do you understand the short- and long-term risks of living in this alternative manner?

The evaluation process may begin with the diagnostic criteria for gender dysphoria, but this can be indirectly accomplished by asking about the evolution of gender identity, orientation, and intention as the person remembers that development over time. Since the onset of gender dysphoria may occur from early childhood to the senior years, patients may or may not know much about their sexual identity components.

We also want to identify associated mental and physical ailments. When we ask about the family, we want to know about all family members' attitudes about the new identity. This includes spouses, children, siblings, and parents. Some of the patients grossly overestimate the degree of support within their families. It is important to see the parents of children and adolescents.

These tasks of the evaluation expose us to the personality traits of the patient as we try to assess the decision-making capacity.[20] We want to know what the patient thinks are the benefits and risks of transition. At the end of the evaluation, we need to determine with the patient what he or she wants to do next. Shall we continue to try to define the reasons for the repudiation of your gender identity in the hope that you may find another path for yourself? Shall we first attend to the associated psychiatric and medical problems before you decide what path to take? Shall we do nothing but wait and see how this plays out over time and have another meeting in 3–6 months? Shall we move ahead immediately with transition and hormones or surgery?

Informed Consent

There are three categories of risks that ideally the patient understands and agrees to undertake.[21] The age, education, and mental health of the patient shape the decision as to whether or not the patient actually grasps the risks that are inherent in social transition, hormonal therapy, genital surgery, mastectomy, augmentation mammoplasty, and various other head and neck surgeries. All mental health professionals and physicians carry an ethical responsibility to convey the risks and ways to minimize them. In mathematical terms, the actual risks range from 100% to uncertain. Considering that mental health professionals have been involved in assessment of suitability for reassignment for about 50 years, it is a little embarrassing that the negative consequences of transitioning have not been better articulated.

A. *Biological risks* include infertility in both biological male and female trans individuals; impaired sexual functional capacity among males taking estrogenic compounds; increased sexual drive in those taking testosterone; shortened life expectancy; and the fact that in a biological sense, sex cannot be changed (only gender can).
B. *Social risks* include emotional distancing and isolation from family members; exchange of friends for those real and virtual friends in the trans community; a greatly diminished pool of individuals who are willing to sustain

an intimate physical and loving relationship; and social and vocational discrimination.

C. *Mental health risks* include deflection from personal developmental challenges that would otherwise be mastered at appropriate times; eventual feeling of inauthenticity in the established role as a member of the other gender or as a nonbinary person; demoralization with new or exacerbation of psychiatric symptoms; heightened risk of suicide; and continuing outsider status.

All of these more or less separate risks need to be seriously considered, planned for in order to avoid, or made personally unimportant in the future. (To take but one example of the last mentioned, a 16-year-old may insist that he or she does not and never will want to be a parent so that infertility is of no concern. "Anyway, I can always adopt or be a step- or foster parent." Professionals wonder if the dismissal of infertility will be as glib and remorseless at age 30.)

Based on existing social research, it has recently been reported that gender minority persons, compared with the general population, are more likely to live in poverty (29% vs. 12%), be unemployed (15% vs. 5%), be a victim of intimate-partner violence (24% vs. 18%), have attempted suicide (40% vs. 4.6%), have experienced severe psychological stress in the previous month (39% vs. 5%), and have HIV (1.4% vs. 0.3%).[22] These health disparities are used to point out how ill equipped many physicians are in understanding the health care needs of trans people and what must be done to make health care environments more trans welcoming. Authors do not use these and other data about the psychiatric and social patterns of trans people (a vulnerable population group) to raise the question of whether it is a wise decision to repudiate one's originally assigned gender. That seems to be politically unacceptable. Some assume that trans individuals are biologically created. I think the negative outcomes that are known not only should be a clarion call for better medical education of health professionals[23] but also should be built in to the informed consent process. The fact that clinicians are correct in their view that some people do fine in their new gendered adaptations does not erase the numerous parameters that suggest that many others do not.

Ethical Tensions

You are familiar with five ethical principles:

1. Above all do no harm (to the body, to physiology, to life expectancy, to mental life).
2. Act in the best interest of the patient (in the short and long term).

3. Ensure justice in the delivery of care (the poor deserve the same excellent treatment as the wealthy).
4. Maintain respect for patient autonomy. (When established science does not dictate the therapeutic path to take, the adult patient should have the major decision on how to proceed.)
5. Base clinical decisions on science, not personal politics.

The reason that many professionals are uneasy in working with this sexual minority group is that these ethical principles often clash with one another to distress the professional. Should respect for patient autonomy be the most important guideline when patients do not seem able to tolerate knowing the risks or think that the risks are not relevant in their case? Should acting in the patient's best interest to relieve incongruence through immediate transition with hormone administration[24] be the right thing to do when it means rejection from the family and new severe depression in the parents, spouse, or children? You can see why the pediatrician, endocrinologist, primary care physician, or surgeon wants a letter giving them the recommendation to proceed ("The mental health professional said it was indicated").

Embracing Controversy

I do not want to pretend that our professional activities are heavily based on science, because science is rooted in skepticism and our differing mental health professions are based on many ideological assumptions. WPATH wants professionals to advocate for the treatments that patients desire. Science advances by asking for proof. It is well acquainted with distinctions between short- and long-term benefits. Advocacy ignores evidence that does not support its cause.

When topics are recognized as controversial, particularly when they are passionately so, it means that individuals with a different set of assumptions reach opposite conclusions. One group is typically not entirely right or wrong. What the minimal requirements are for an initial mental health evaluation and who is qualified to perform it are controversial. The field of medicine is used to unanswered controversial questions. It is passionately controversial whether a child of 11 should be placed on puberty-blocking hormones, because this immediately stirs up ethical concerns. We are aware that certain ideas are socially acceptable even though they are far from scientifically established. This is the situation with the biological origins of homosexuality, for example. It is controversial that gender identity and orientation are two entirely separate unrelated aspects of sexual identity. Although this idea is often disproven in the lives of trans individuals, it continues to be promulgated by WPATH and professional organizations that derive their policies from this organization.

Perhaps we cannot wait until science answers the questions that clinicians raise. In the meantime, we have to make decisions with and sometimes for our patients. I suggest that these often-difficult judgments be made knowing full well what is controversial and why.[6] Sadly, in this arena, there is a tendency to tyranny. It is as though "If you don't agree with me, you are incompetent." Nonetheless, the gender revolution has made for some fascinating discoveries about the pathways to human happiness. Do not shy away from it; there is too much to learn.

Now let's shift our focus to a more subtle, related matter.

The Therapeutic Sexual Identity Alignment

Listed below are some of the combinations of sexual identities when therapists and their patients do their work together:

1. Both are heterosexual.
2. Both are gay.
3. Both are sexual minorities but of differing types.
4. The therapist is homosexual, and the patient is heterosexual.
5. The therapist is heterosexual, and the patient is homosexual.
6. The therapist is trans (often a nonpsychiatric physician), and the client is not.
7. The therapist is atypically masculine or feminine appearing, and the patient is trans, lesbian, bisexual, or gay.
8. The therapist works in a setting for care of sexual minorities.

Theoretically, aspects of a therapist's sexual identity should not be an issue. After all, the patients are here for their issues in order to benefit from the therapist's skills, knowledge, and compassionate understanding. The manner of most lesbian and gay therapists does not suggest their orientation, but some patients have the capacity to accurately identify one's orientation ("gaydar"). This may or may not create a disruption of the therapeutic alliance.

Who the therapist is has great meaning to those who seek our care. Many heterosexual clients may be uncomfortable knowing that their therapists are not. They may make many unfounded assumptions about the therapist and simply refuse to have a second visit. This is often the explanation for some unexplained no-shows for second appointments to competent therapists. Just a few patients in our clinic have called over the years and asked to be reassigned for this reason.

Many individuals struggling with their own sexual identity issue are pleased to have a therapist whom they perceive to be gay or lesbian. Without discussing the therapist's perceived orientation, the patient feels more comfortable and is encouraged that a better life is possible. "My therapist seems to have it all together." Later in the therapy the positive meanings of the therapist's orientation may emerge, but not in a disruptive way.

When a patient calls an institution for assignment to a therapist, the intake professional maintains the potential therapist's privacy by not revealing any personal information such as specific age, marital status, ethnicity, orientation, or race. Sometimes callers specify wanting a lesbian, gay, trans-friendly, or trans-competent therapist. The last two terms generally mean a therapist who will immediately support their wishes. Institutions will not readily reveal a therapist's orientation without the therapist's consent. The intake professional tries to match the caller with a therapist primarily on the goodness of fit between the reason for seeking assistance and the therapists' experience or qualifications. The therapist's sexual identity should not be the primary determinant in the assignment. Nonetheless, the caller's request cannot be ignored; it is further explored.

Once the relationship begins, the patient in any form of psychotherapy will have many impressions of the therapist, will be curious, and will experience many feelings about the therapist that are not shared in therapy. A seemingly innocuous question may arise: "Are you married?" Most of us have been taught not to directly answer such an inquiry. Rather, knowing that there is something important lurking behind it, we ask, "Can you tell me what is behind the question?" Sometimes the person will directly ask, "Are you gay?" or "Are you heterosexual?" I suggest that you start by asking, "Can you tell me what is prompting the question?" Then, depending on the answer, "What do you feel about the possibility that I am?" Let the patient continue to talk. Eventually, you can note, "You haven't spoken yet about your identity. This seems like a good opportunity for us to talk about that." If you do reveal your orientation, please feel free to inquire over time how the patient thinks and feels about it now. This is particularly relevant if the patient soon thereafter seems to be resistant or uncooperative with the tasks of treatment.

Occasionally, when someone asks me an "innocuous" personal question, I offer a deal. "I will answer your question, if you still desire an answer, after we explore your question in detail." Often, after the mirror is held up to the patient's motives for asking, the patient is no longer interested in the answer. A therapist will, of course, not be able to handle all such moments with aplomb. Even so, we can quickly recover by reminding ourselves that therapy is about the patient's struggles. "Enough about me. Let's return to you"

When dealing with any patient with sexual dysfunction, clinicians are correct to wonder how the patient's symptoms relate to their sexual identities.

Is the symptom a product of a struggle within the patient's sexual identity mosaic or is it irrelevant? Do not think that a married apparently heterosexual person could not be having a struggle with one of the elements of sexual identity. With sexual minority patients, the therapist must be careful not to too quickly conclude that the patient's sexual dysfunction is due to conflicts about sexual identity. Sexual minority patients have the same sexual dysfunction problems as those seen in the larger heteronormative community. Yes, there is more substance abuse, alcoholism, and suicide in minority communities, but most of these individuals are mentally well people grappling with the same issues that those with conventional identities are: love, work, social life, family of origin obligations, physical health, and, of course, performance anxiety.

In the literature of sexual identity variations, there is a strong focus on internalized self-hatred and the coming-out process. All therapists should be able to recognize and discuss the arduous prolonged process of coming out to oneself, friends, siblings, parents, and extended family, and to the workplace. Some patients may want guidance on how to deal with family members, not only how and when to tell them but also how to regard family members' initial and subsequent reactions. It may be that gay and lesbian therapists are more sensitive to these processes and may spend more time trying to attenuate any residual internalized homophobia (or trans phobia) and helping with intrafamilial communication. This is one of the reasons that many sexual minority patients prefer a therapist from their sexual community. This reminds me that the gamut of 24 aspects of identity of the therapist outlined in this chapter may shape the processes and content of what comes into focus during our work together.

References

1. Byne W, Karasic DH, Coleman E, et al: Gender dysphoria in adults: an overview and primer for psychiatrists. Transgend Health 3(1):57–73, 2018
2. FightingToGetHerBack: Why I supported my autistic daughter's social transition to a man. Posted June 7, 2018. Available at: https://4thwavenow.com/?s=Why+I+supported+my+autistic+daughter%E2%80%99s+social+transition+to+a+man&submit=Search. Accessed June 7, 2018.
3. Levine SB: Transitioning back to maleness. Arch Sex Behav 47(4):1295–1300, 2018
4. Litmann L: Rapid-onset gender dysphoria in adolescents and young adults: a study of parental reports. PLoS One Aug 16;13(8):e0202330, 2018
5. Drescher J, Haller E, APA Caucus of Lesbian, Gay and Bisexual Psychiatrists: Position statement on discrimination against transgender and gender variant individuals. Am J Psychiatry 169:8, August 2012

6. Mayer LS, McHugh PR: Sexuality and gender: findings from the biological, psychological, and social sciences. The New Atlantis: A Journal of Technology & Society 50:10–143, 2016

7. Corradi RB: Psychiatry professor: 'Transgenderism' is mass hysteria similar to 1980s-era junk science. The Federalist November 17, 2016. Available at: https://thefederalist.com/2016/11/17/psychiatry-professor-transgenderismmass-hysteria-similar-1980s-era-junk-science/#.WDyzMzIVavU.email. Accessed January 2, 2017.

8. Dreger AD: Galileo's Middle Finger: Heretics, Activists, and One Scholar's Search for Justice. New York, Penguin Press, 2015

9. Hayes M: Doctor fired from gender identity clinic says he feels 'vindicated' after CAMH apology, settlement. Toronto Globe and Mail, October 7, 2018. Available at: https://www.theglobeandmail.com/canada/toronto/article-doctor-fired-from-gender-identity-clinic-says-he-feels-vindicated.

10. American Psychiatric Association. Diagnostic and Statistical Manual of Mental Disorders, 5th Edition. Arlington, VA, American Psychiatric Publishing, 2013

11. James SE, Herman JL, Rankin S, et al: The Report of the 2015 U.S. Transgender Survey. Washington, DC, National Center for Transgender Equality, 2016. Available at: https://www.transequality.org/sites/default/files/docs/USTS-Full-Report-FINAL.PDF. Accessed October 10, 2018.

12. Strang JF, Janssen A, Tishelman A, et al: Revisiting the link: evidence of the rates of autism in studies of gender diverse individuals. J Am Acad Child Adolesc Psychiatry 57(11):885–887, 2018

13. Mathews T, Holt V, Sahin S, et al: Gender dysphoria in looked-after and adopted young people in a gender identity development practice. Clin Child Psychol Psychiatry 24(1):112–128, 2018

14. Osborne C, Lawrence AA: Male prison inmates with gender dysphoria: when is sex reassignment surgery appropriate? Arch Sex Behavior 45(7):1649–1663, 2016

15. Meyer-Bahlburg HF, Baratz Dalke K, Berenbaum SA, et al. Gender assignment, reassignment and outcome in disorders of sex development: update of the 2005 Consensus Conference. Horm Res Paediatr 85(2):112–118, 2016

16. Grant JM, Mottet LA, Tanis J, et al: Injustice at Every Turn: A Report of the National Transgender Discrimination Survey. Washington, DC, National Center for Transgender Equality, 2010. Available at www.thetaskforce.org/static_html/downloads/reports/reports/ntds_full.pdf. Accessed October 10, 2018.

17. Dragon CN, Guerino P, Ewald E, Laffan AM: Transgender Medicare beneficiaries and chronic conditions: exploring fee-for-service claims data. LGBT Health. 4(6):404–411, 2017

18. Dheyne C, Lichtenstein P, Boman M, et al: Long-term follow-up of transsexual person undergoing sex reassignment surgery: cohort study in Sweden. PLoS One Feb 22;6(2):e16885, 2011

19. Byne W, Bradley S, Coleman E, et al; Report of the APA Task Force on Treatment of Gender Identity Disorder. Am J Psychiatry 169(8, suppl):1–35, August 2012

20. Levine SB: Ethical concerns about the emerging treatment paradigms for gender dysphoria. J Sex Marital Ther 44(1):29–44, 2018

21. Levine SB: Informed consent for transgender patients. J Sex Marital Ther 2018 Dec 22:1–12, 2018 (Epub ahead of print)

22. Liszewski W, Peebles K, Yeung H, Arron S: Persons of nonbinary gender—awareness, visibility, and health disparities. N Engl J Med 379(25):2391–2393, 2018
23. Ard KL, Keuroghlian AS: Training in sexual and gender health—expanding education to reach all clinicians. N Engl J Med 379(25):2388–2391, 2018
24. Samuels J, Keisling M: The anti-trans memo—abandoning doctors and patients. N Engl J Med 380(2):111–113, 2019

8 | Another Barrier to Loving: Paraphilia

Part I: Love

After specializing in clinical aspects of sexuality for 20 years, I began to develop the conviction that these problems were part of a rarely clinically discussed transcendent process called *love*. Love is ubiquitously referenced in the culture in song and stories, yet it rarely finds its way to mental health professionals' discussions other than in sentences such as "She doesn't love him anymore." I eventually decided to learn more about love. At this point in my life, I am sure love is not one thing and that, like identity, it evolves. Felt and expressed love in adolescence, charming though it is, is not the same as felt and expressed love 40 years later. This is not insightful, even if it is not usually put into words.

As I came to define aspects of love, I began to believe that I better understood sexual dysfunctions as they occurred in patients of any sexual identity configuration. Knowing that the phenomenon of love can be described in at least nine ways and that each of the delineations undergoes evolution from one phase of life to another, it is not surprising how varied are the barriers to feeling and expressing love. In this chapter, I want to consider nine ways of defining love with you in preparation for thinking about just one category of the barriers to loving. Paraphilias, variations in the third aspect of sexual identity (i.e., intention), like the other two (i.e., gender identity and orientation), are also a politically charged subject (see Chapter 7). Some of the paraphilias are criminal behaviors. Pedophilia is the universally repudiated one. Most, however, are private acts that enhance the person's ability to be aroused to orgasm. Sadomasochism with a like-minded cooperative partner seems to pose no issue for mental health professionals, except when an accident occurs.

The problem posed by many paraphilias is their impact on wary partners who find it difficult to bond or sustain an attachment through sex under such conditions. To better appreciate how these variations in the intention component of identity interfere with love, I want to first share a little about love itself.

Love Is Not One Thing*

An Ambition

Love is an ambition to attain a lasting state of interpersonal harmony that will ensure enough contentment that the person will be able to focus on other important matters such as raising healthy children, having a good job or successful career, or enjoying life. It can also be conventionally conceptualized as the ambition to live a life characterized by mutual respect, behavioral reliability, enjoyment of each other, sexual pleasure and fidelity, psychological intimacy, and a comfortable balance of individuality and couplehood. Or, if you prefer, love's ambition is the hope of finding a partner who will accompany, assist, emotionally stabilize, and enrich us as we evolve, mature, and cope with life's demands. However defined, the ambition has two faces: to be loved and to be able to love another.

A Deal

During courtship at any time in life, people ask themselves, "What will this relationship do for me?" They are trying to decide whether to continue with the relationship—to accept the deal that apparently is being offered. This question is applied to social, economic, aesthetic, recreational, sexual, medical, and, for older people or those with a serious illness, time-to-death contexts. "Shall I commit myself to this person" is a decision made as a result of a vetting process, a process that may be made just once, early in life, or multiple times, after a relationship ends by breakup, divorce, or death. Shall I accept the deal? When accepted, the new arrangement represents a satisfactory exchange of assets, despite recognized drawbacks. An asset can be material, a person's capacities, beauty, athleticism, intellect, social connections, family structure, and so on. When parents arrange a marriage, they are focused on assets and their couple's likely compatibility. The children better understand that their emotional acceptance of the deal must occur after the wedding. Arranged marriages are a reminder of the cultural influences on sexual behaviors.

---

*This section is adapted from my earlier book *Demystifying Love*.[1]

An Attachment

Once the deal is largely worked out in the partners' minds, they weave their psyches together and begin to feel a hunger to be with the other more. They think of themselves as belonging with, and to, the other. A new form of identity emerges, couplehood, though not necessarily at the same rate or to the same extent for each partner. Sexual activities facilitate the mental process of attachment, which in turn induces strong motivation to attain love's ambitions. Love as an attachment is often referred to as a *bond*.

A Moral Commitment

The rituals that sanctify marriage emphasize love as a moral commitment. Clergy teach the couple that love is a commitment to try to realize love's grand ambitions. The ceremony officially raises the bar of expectations; spouses are expected to honor their vows. Whether religious or secular, the ceremony instantly restructures life and generates a new set of obligations in their own and their community's minds. Those who are serious about their vows will feel painful, persistent guilt when they contemplate extramarital affairs and divorce. The moral nature of the commitment is more excruciatingly felt when unhappily married parents grapple with the agonizing dilemma of their commitment to provide their children with two live-in parents and the wish to be free of unhappiness with their partner.

A Management Process

Many of the positive and, particularly, negative mental processes involved in loving remain private from the partner. We wisely do not share too much of our anger and disappointment about our partner. We intuitively realize that our partners need the illusion that we do not struggle to love them. Love requires day-to-day work to remain prudent about what one says, to continue to be diplomatic about how one says it, to maintain perspective about the bigger things in one's life, and to prevent the partner from realizing what is actually transpiring within one's mind. Each partner's relationship is a separate subjective state and process; this is why I emphasize that in every marriage there are two marriages. Continuing love represents mutual good management. The mental struggle to maintain cooperative, kind behaviors exists in the happily married as well as among those in distressing relationships.

A Force of Nature

Love casts our fates together, organizes reproduction, and remains vital to our adult growth and development and to the maturation of our children. Nature acts on us without a constant awareness of its presence. Love is most pleasingly discussed at the beginning of relationships, but it can also be seen during later years when people stay together because they have always been together, even though the forces that brought them together have long since vanished. Older people who are not delighted with their partners often recognize that their mate is now an inextricable part of themselves and that they can never be psychologically free of the partner. Nature, the underlying biological force that brought them together socially, gave them culturally approved tasks that kept them together, and now, having slowly attenuated their capacities, has had its way with them.

A Transient Emotional State

Love is not *a* feeling. It is a combination of three, and sometimes more, feelings: pleasure, interest, and appreciation. For many people, the periodic experience of these feelings is a prerequisite for sexual pleasure. The words *feeling* and *emotion* are not synonyms. A feeling is a simple experience of sadness, anger, disappointment, aversion, pleasure, or interest. The capacity to have such feelings is a human characteristic. An emotion consists of two or more simultaneous feelings. One or more affects are our first warning system for the changes in our external and interpersonal environment. Anything important to us typically creates an array of feelings. In addition, we have feelings about our feelings. For example, a young child experiences envy. Some children are taught that envy is wrong. "You should not be envious!" The next time this simple feeling arises, it invokes anxiety, guilt, or shame. The child now has the emotion of envy-anxiety or envy-guilt. In this way one person's feeling may be unencumbered, while another with the same feeling experiences a more complicated emotion. Different cultures may teach different attitudes toward basic feelings.

The emotions of love are typically complicated. Feeling intense pleasure, appreciation, and interest in a potential new partner quickly stimulates some internal reaction to this incipient love. It may be positive or negative depending on the person's past or current life. *Love* is the label we give to a range of transient emotional experiences. When individuals can sincerely state that they recurrently feel love for their partners, they are likely referencing their experiences of interest, pleasure, motivation to behave sexually with the partner, caring for or devotion to the partner, and the conviction that their lives will be better with than without the partner. Any one of these experiences may be labeled *love* at times.

An Illusion

We want to think positively about love, to believe in it as a concept, to think that our partner's love for us is constant and that we love our partner. In order to maintain these beliefs, we need to create certain distortions both for ourselves and for our partners. Love as an illusion refers to the fact that we create love by internal private processes, maintain it by prudent diplomatic dishonesties, and can lose it for our partner without the partner knowing it. Love as an illusion only means that self-perceptions as loving and as beloved can prove to be inaccurate. It also means that society, through its educational and religious institutions, through its celebrations of love in song, and through its academic discourses on the topics, fosters simplistic notions about love that encourage us to behave as though we all know what it is. Many people privately wonder what person-to-person love is.

A Conversational Stop Sign

Many patients are baffled about or hard put to explain why they love their partner in the face of the partner's destructive behavior. Their reticence can be an unwillingness to answer the question, but it can also signal an unwillingness to think about the question. It often means, "I don't want to pursue the subject further!" The explanation people use when they do not want to examine their motivations is love. "Because I love him (her)" ends the inquiry.

A Brief Summary

None of these nine definitions indicate that love is static. Love is an active evolving mental process. It may begin with an attraction and then be followed by elaboration in imagination and, later, by the pair's actual interactions. When these processes go well, the wonderful process of falling in love results. When both realize that they are their beloved's beloved, a radical transformation of their psyches occurs. Each feels pleasure, interest, appreciation, sexual desire, and devotion, and believes that "I will be better off with this person." These six aspects of felt new love might be restated as the possession of psychological intimacy, intense sexual interest, and commitment. Each person attempts to realize the long-term ambitions of love. Being in love in this manner is relatively short-lived because the newly mutually affirmed couple must take on life functioning both as one entity and as two persons. They then face the rest of life trying to remain respectful, caring, sexual, supportive, and kind. Staying in love is the great challenge. It tends to be accomplished by those who can largely refrain from hostility, negotiate disagreements, put the needs of their partners first at times, remain genuine, and maintain their perspective about what is important. Staying in love is a management process. People are not equally skilled at it.

In an ideal circumstance being in love enables the couple to deepen their bond by what they share sexually. What they reveal to each other in their affective processes during sex is highly valued by both. While couples who spend 50 or 60 years together after such a beginning are likely to end up with a limited or nonexistent sexual life together, they may say that they love each other more than ever. Wonderful sex may be more important to young adulthood and the middle years than in the last portions of life. Realized sexual pleasures cement the bonding process of love, but these decades of experiences then become the vehicle for the emotionally stabilizing sense that I love and am loved, in my partner's unique way. Sex becomes far less necessary.[*]

Sexuality, dysfunctional or not, has different characteristics at different stages of life. The contexts for understanding sexual concerns are childhood, adolescence, young single adulthood, attached, parenthood, early midlife, perimenopause, menopause, early aging, and advanced aging. Anywhere in this developmental sequence serious illness may occur, which typically changes sexual expression. Serious illness may cause adults to define for themselves whether they still love each other. The other factor that routinely disrupts sexual expression is relationship deterioration followed by breakup, divorce, or death. The treatment of a sexual dysfunction such as anorgasmia or erectile dysfunction is undertaken by first considering the patient's age and stage in life, relationship status, physical health, and mental capacities. Mental health clinicians cannot say that the treatment of X is Y.

The end of partnered sexual life in a long-married couple does not usually create a request for medical or psychological care. The exception is a married elderly man who wants a PDE-5 inhibitor drug to use with a paramour. He may initially imply it is to use at home, but what he tells you about their long asexual adjustment may prompt you to ask about another partner. The elderly who will more often seek your assistance are those who are beginning with a new partner after a long period of not having any partner sex. Gynecologists and primary care physicians tend to see women in such situations, and psychiatrists tend to see their male patients who are divorced or widowed.

Those who more routinely seek our professional assistance are young and middle-age individuals and couples who have not had sex together for a long time. Our role is to understand what undermined their interest and ability to be together, beginning with each partner's perspectives. It is a luxury for us when they agree on what ended their sexual life together. We can help them express their emotions and personal meanings about the event and in doing so reestablish psychological intimacy. This therapist-catalyzed state of

---

[*]Even so, mental health professionals are consulted by individuals and couples because of difficulties maintaining intercourse, typically because of painful intercourse from an atrophic vagina or an erectile dysfunction in the face of chronic illness. You should know that some couples continue to make love with the capacities that they have.[2] Painful intercourse and erectile dysfunction tend to shift mutual orgasmic attainment to oral sex, for instance.

knowing one is understood and accepted without censure motivates the couple's return to lovemaking. Concepts about love can be useful. These individuals demonstrate to us that love can be a process of connection, disconnection, reconnection, disconnection, and reconnection. Although I do not know what is discussed about love in my colleagues' offices, I have long noticed how valuable my explanations of the different meanings of love are to my patients.

Part II: The Paraphilias

Eight specific paraphilic disorders are listed in DSM-5 along with categories called other and unspecified: voyeuristic disorder, exhibitionistic disorder, frotteuristic disorder, sexual masochism disorder, sexual sadism disorder, pedophilic disorder, fetishistic disorder, and transvestic disorder.[3] The additional categories could possibly contain over 250 esoterically named relatively unique intentions.[4] In the past, paraphilias were labeled sexual deviance or perversion. Today, paraphilias are seen as part of human sexual diversity. A paraphilia is not diagnosed as a disorder unless the patient is over age 18; has strong recurrent urges, fantasies, or behaviors that have been present for at least 6 months; or has acted upon these desires with a nonconsenting person. These characteristics are not conspicuously relevant to victimless fetishism and transvestism. If the person has not victimized another and is not personally distressed by their intention, and the behavior does not interfere with social, vocational, or other areas of functioning (left undefined in DSM-5), the pattern is simply described as a "paraphilia." It implies no mental illness.

Many of the individuals who qualify for a DSM-5 paraphilic disorder are seen in forensic settings after they have been identified as having victimized others. They are evaluated prior to adjudication. They may obtain some form of treatment in prison or be remanded to be in treatment in lieu of prison. Outpatient therapists tend to encounter paraphilia when evaluating men and women who have limited sexual desire, arousal, or orgasmic capacities with a partner unless a paraphilic fantasy or behavior is part of the lovemaking. Wives are often the ones who initiate the appointments. The sexual dysfunction often remains enigmatic until the therapist inquires about fantasies during the course of asking about the erotic and behavioral expression of sexual identity components.

So what does paraphilia have to do with love?

A man with a lingerie fetish buys his partner underwear, which pleases both of them until she begins to sense that he is more interested in touching her breast and genital coverings than what is beneath them. When she is naked, he is unexcitable; when she is clothed in the underwear he has chosen, he is eagerly potent.

You can substitute many things in this vignette, such as a high-heeled shoe, pantyhose, an article of leather, hair, or animal fur. These inanimate things are what enable his arousal. Some partners, female and male, regard this lightly, "Everyone is a little kinky, you know. What's the big deal?" They tend to sustain the sexual relationship until they, too, tire of the imposition of the inanimate object. The man typically has a masturbatory life that integrates the fetish without any distress.

Some paraphilias are less likely to sustain partner sexual life for a long period of time. They sometimes are the reasons for ending a marriage.

> A 49-year-old man claimed that he had not been sexually unusual until he visited a sex club in college. Since then, he has not been able to free himself from the memories of watching people in various sex acts. These images populate his masturbation fantasies and sex with his wife. After his children left for college, he began to pressure his wife to have sex with someone else while he watched. She thought it ridiculous. "That's sick!" He persisted and after several years of coercion, she assented as long as she could approve the man. This pleased him greatly. He was grateful to her and wanted to repeat it. She did so with another consenting man. With the third experience, her enjoyment increased. She started to have a clandestine affair and then refused to acquiesce to her husband's wishes. He became enraged. She soon changed her mind about her affair and began to hate herself and her husband for this process. During her work with a therapist, she decided to end the marriage. She told her therapist that throughout their years together, she acquiesced to his domination. "He always pushed me. I've had enough. He ruined everything. I'm ashamed of myself."

You can also substitute several other behaviors for this man's wish to see his wife with another. Making up stories about having sex with others, telling of past sexual encounters with men or women or both, and coercing a wife to wrestle or physically fight another woman are a few examples. What DSM-5 calls "or other important areas of functioning" I think really means the impact on the sexual partner. When I wonder why this recurring consequence of paraphilia on partners was omitted from the criteria, I remind myself that nosology development involves stakeholders and social movements.[5] The DSM-5 paraphilia section was composed in the face of paraphilic stakeholders who did not want their private consenting acts to be classified in the same way as pedophilic acts were. They did not want to be viewed as having a mental disorder. The committee listened and separated paraphilias from paraphilic disorders. This was in keeping with a larger movement to depathologize all sexual diversities.[6] DSM-5 emphasized that an individual has the paraphilia; the criteria are based on the consequences for him or her. Regardless, paraphilias often have a powerful inhibiting impact on the partner.

One way of looking at the pathway to paraphilia is an individual's unconscious creative response to something that overwhelmed or traumatized him or her at an earlier period of life. This is one explanation for why there are so many distinct paraphilic preferences. The partner has had no such life experience and has not eroticized the same events. Adapting to a partner's paraphilic interest is something one may have to do for love. But sadly, the self-centeredness, drivenness, and coerciveness of the paraphilia interfere with the capacity to love because, like the wife of the man with a women's underwear fetish, she realizes that the sexual interest is in the fetish, not her. A person can do this for a partner, but often not indefinitely, because it is not arousing to her and her attitude toward it may change or fluctuate. Both men and women, heterosexual and homosexual in orientation, want to be the object of their partner's sexual desire. The inanimate nature of the arousing interest not only is insulting but also adds to the idea that the partner is a strange quirky person.

> DEBRA: You desire my long hair, not me!
> PAUL: It is *your* hair I love to touch!
> DEBRA: But you would have an orgasm touching any woman's hair.
> PAUL: Well, I admit that's probably true, but you're my only partner and I love you.
> DEBRA: And you got so depressed after I cut my hair short. What a reason to get depressed!
> PAUL: I felt you had rejected me.
> DEBRA: I got tired of the time my hair took every day. I wanted a new look, and I wondered if you would still want to have sex with me. It was only then that your trouble being hard began.

> JOHN: I don't want to play rough with you anymore.
> SUE: Why not, it turns me on.
> JOHN: It doesn't turn me on. It makes me feel like I'm not important. It makes me feel depraved.
> SUE: But I love you. I want you to spank me, no one else.
> JOHN: Do you realize you continually want more, to push me further?
> SUE: I'm sorry. I'm not the only woman like this.
> JOHN: You're the only one in my life, and I don't like me for doing this to you.

The most common paraphilia seen among women in my and my colleagues' practices is sexual masochistic disorder. A woman can be introduced to this world of pleasure through pain via a partner or can entice a partner to treat her in a dominating manner. "Pull my hair, hit me across the face, whip me, etc." In coupled masochistic women, there are those who play the dominant and the submissive roles at various times and those who only want to be spanked, beaten, humiliated, bound, asphyxiated, or caused pain, or made to feel submissive or degraded in some other way. Clinicians tend to see masochistic women in other circumstances—usually depression. I have known of four women who lost their lives from masochistic behaviors, three who were accidently asphyxiated and one who was accidently dropped from a window when her partner's grip on a rope slipped. After such deaths, their male partners may be seen for evaluation prior to adjudication. One can only wonder how many masochistic women obtain treatment for depression without sharing their masochistic desires. Here is an exception, although the patient did not persist in therapy:

> A physician retired at age 45 after she was put on a leave of absence because of depression. She eventually sought psychotherapy after she went to a sex club in another city on several occasions where she arranged to be suspended naked from the ceiling so that anyone at the club could penetrate her anus or vagina with a finger or dildo. "I know this is sick, but I found it pleasing to be helpless, although after an hour in suspension I was very uncomfortable and had trouble feeling my legs."

The lesser forms of submissive masochism are probably the most common as women experiment with pain and anoxia as enhancements of pleasure. There are organizations devoted to safe domination and submission and many guidebooks. The keys are consent and trust; when the submissive signals stop, the behavior immediately ends. When men are masochistic and their partners want no part of this behavior, these men often find their way to a dominatrix who sells her services in her "dungeon." As with the masochistic women, we only get to see these men when something goes wrong, such as when self-tied ligatures cause bodily harm, a horrified wife discovers her husband's use of a dominatrix, or a man seeks help for depression that has not been improved by his foray into masochism. Most therapists only get occasional clinical glimpses of sadomasochism.

> A 76-year-old athletic independent woman, who has been asexually married to a chronically ill man since age 50, years ago decided that fidelity made little sense for her. Her husband was sexually nervous when he occasionally initiated sex. She consulted with me 2 years into her marriage about her sexual disappointment, seeking a means to negotiate their dramatically different energy levels: she who embraces adventure and novelty; he who wants to stay at home and check the stock market most of the day. Periodically over the years she returned to talk with me. Much more recently, she returned to see me to discuss her recent lover who responded to her website ad. The charming man in his 60s eventually explained to her after their lunch and un-self-centered sex that he wanted to be her slave. He would do anything she wanted to do sexually and anything she commanded him to do outside the bedroom. Never having heard of this, she was intrigued and found him to be a compliant, dutiful, pleasure-giving lover who only wanted from her clarity about what his queen

desired. He once suggested he would be happy to dress as a woman if she desired. "Anything you want." He never made any demands. She was happy to allow him to do errands and cook for her when she was apart from her husband. This lasted for several months until she tired of sex with a servant. She was hoping to have a permanent paramour, but the lack of his independent self began to bore her. He was heartbroken and offered to resume anytime "Momma" desired.

Single Individuals With Paraphilia

Many of the adult voyeurs, exhibitionists, pedophiles, fetishists, masochists, and frotteurs, and some of the transvestites, who will come to your clinical attention will be socially isolated individuals who seem profoundly unready to enter into a relationship with another person. A few married somehow, even had a child, but throughout the marriage have avoided emotional, social, and sexual contact with their partner. They prefer their paraphilic behaviors. It is hard to imagine that these men and, occasionally, women are able to participate in love as has been described. In these situations, paraphilia is not the most conspicuous diagnosis. Instead, alcoholism, periodic psychosis, substance abuse, posttraumatic stress disorder, social anxiety, autism, or intellectual disability is also present. Your treatment of the paraphilia will likely begin with taking into account these other features.

Specialists in treating paraphilias rely heavily on group therapies that teach social skills and end social isolation, and medication to help with underlying psychiatric conditions.[4,7] Patients are encouraged to seek substance abuse treatment. There is an early indication that the drug naloxone, which diminishes craving for alcohol, also can reduce paraphilic drivenness. If this proves true in a clinical trial or with more extensive clinical experience, professionals may feel more optimistic about investing in these individuals.

Thwarting Love

Immersion in clinical sexuality endlessly demonstrates behaviors that thwart the ambition to love. The specific symptomatic mechanisms, such as low desire, excessive motivation for sex, sex of an unwanted kind, anorgasmia, pain and fear of penetration, and unreliable erections, all carry negative potentials. Outcomes include ending partner sex, being unfaithful, resentfully increasingly relying on masturbation, and ending the relationship. Therapists rarely get to see couples who have happily integrated a paraphilia into their lives. There is then no reason to consult us about sex.

A successful happily married businessman and beloved father, an entrepreneur who was widely known for his philanthropic involvements, developed a pituitary prolactinoma, which presented with loss of sexual desire and erectile dysfunction. In the process of discovering his problem, which was medically treated and restored his sexual function, he related to me how he and his wife preferred to initiate sex. It began with a ritual that had been repeated for over 40 years. He dressed in a raincoat and knocked on the front door. His wife, clad in a nightgown, asked, "Who is there?" "The Fuller Brush man" (a company that sold brushes door to door in the 1940s and 1950s), he would reply. His wife would open the door, and he would express surprise at her sheer nightgown. He would then show her he was wearing nothing under his raincoat. Giggling, they would move to the bedroom.

It is refreshing to learn that some couples do find compatibility of their erotic stories. In this case the couple acted out their desires to have sex with strangers while in fact affirming their monogamy. I think such stories are important for mental health professionals to hear.

Let's remind ourselves that paraphilic interests are but one atypical component of our three-component sexual identity. I have often watched love being thwarted by a major shift in any component of sexual identity as I learn of an incompatibility of a patient's and a partner's sexual identity. For example, when one partner is homosexual and the other is heterosexual, one partner discovers a desire to change gender and the other is content with his or her gender, or one partner has become dominated by a paraphilic interest. Each of these situations creates a barrier to loving. It is difficult to care about the changing partner who has ceased to be the source of pleasure. Resentment and fears of abandonment begin to crowd out committed devotion. The person feels that he or she has been victimized by the partner's sexual identity shift. The one whose sexual identity is changing typically seems increasingly self-centered and unable to consider the needs of the partner and children. The deterioration of love is dangerous to the entire family.

We are not discussing the ordinary human problem of staying in love that challenges trans partners, two gay men, two lesbian women, or a couple that happily practices sadomasochism. These sexual minority couples share many of the same challenges to staying in love that those with conventional sexual identities face. They, too, have problems stemming from their individualities.

You have heard of the occurrence of each of these events. A couple has a happy courtship, marries, has a child or two, and then gets divorced, baffling everyone who knows them. Or 2 months after a seemingly happy wedding, a couple initiates divorce. Does the first example involve growing sexual identity incompatibility as described above? Well, it might. Does the second example involve a discovered sexual dysfunction? Well, it might. But nonsexual processes may create the same scenarios. About the only people who are likely to get enough of the story to explain what happened to them are their trusted therapists with whom they digest their personal misfortunes. Unless you are open to sensitively hearing about their sexual lives, you, too, may be unable to grasp what sullied their ambition to love one another. At this point, you are in position to understand.

References

1. Levine SB: Demystifying Love: Plain Talk for the Mental Health Professional. New York, Routledge, 2006, pp 1–12
2. Kleinplatz PJ, Menard AD, Paquet M, et al: The components of optimal sexuality; a portrait of "great sex." Canadian Journal of Human Sexuality 18(1–2):1–13, 2009
3. American Psychiatric Association: Diagnostic and Statistical Manual of Mental Disorders, 5th Edition. Arlington, VA, American Psychiatric Association, 2013
4. Fedoroff JP: Managing versus successfully treating paraphilic disorders, in Handbook of Clinical Sexuality for Mental Health Professionals, 3rd Edition. Edited by Levine SB, Risen CB, Althof SE. New York, Routledge, 2016, pp 345–361
5. Zucker KJ: The science and politics of diagnosis: reflections on the DSM-5 Work Group on Sexual and Gender Identity Disorders, in Handbook of Clinical Sexuality for Mental Health Professionals, 3rd Edition. Edited by Levine SB, Risen CB, Althof SE. New York, Routledge, 2016, pp 363–368
6. Reed GM, Drescher J, Krueger RB, et al: Disorders related to sexuality and gender identity in the ICD-11: revising the ICD-10 classification based on current scientific evidence, best clinical practices, and human rights considerations. World Psychiatry 5:205–221, 2016
7. Levine SB: Problematic sexual excess. Neuropsychiatry 2(1):1–12, 2012

9 | Sex Is a Psychosomatic Process: Mysteries

We need more people in this field. Newcomers can arrive from many disciplinary backgrounds to choose clinical work, research, education, organizational administration, or some combination of these activities. There will never be a shortage of patients who will seek you out if it is known that there is a reputable professional interested in helping with sexual problems in the community. Some of your colleagues who refer patients to you will eventually become your patients. In a private practice setting, your age, gender, race, ethnicity, orientation, languages spoken, and degree will play a role in why some patients select you, but none of these factors will outweigh your warmth and reputation based on your persistence in trying to help. In institutional settings, patients tend to get assigned to you, but your knowledge, optimism, and professionalism remain vital to the process, whether they return to you, and whether you become known as the institution's resource for sexual problems.

You may have noticed that these chapters are not written as many textbooks are. I have resisted presenting problems in the traditional manner that I so admire for physical diseases—diagnosis, epidemiology, etiology/pathogenesis, treatments and their effectiveness, and unanswered questions. Would that I could present sexual problems in that way. Problems of identity and function are so fundamentally different that I did not want to waste your time with ideas that were not directly useful to understanding sexual histories. I did not want to privilege "disorder" over understanding. There is still much to learn about sexual disorders for which other texts and articles will be helpful. When a disorder is mysterious, as evidenced by our inability to help most of its sufferers or glimpse at its cause, I think of it as an idiopathic syndrome, symptom complex, or disorder.

Most of the authors of textbook chapters and original articles have devoted much of their careers to their subject material. Some of them have had the fortune to see patients with unusual problems that are only occasionally seen and only recently described. Four problems deserve mention if only to label them mysteries.

1. Persistent genital arousal in women
2. Illness after orgasm in men
3. Asexuality in either sex—lifelong absence of sexual desire without a definable orientation
4. Persistent sexual dysfunction long after the offending medication has been metabolized
5. Flooding of enigmatic negative emotions after orgasm in men and women

Calling these problems mysteries does not mean that there are no speculations about how they are produced; it means only that there is considerable uncertainty about cause and treatment. Historically, unexplained problems were assumed to be psychogenic, but the days of separating the mind and body are over. The body is always involved with sex.

Urologists and gynecologists can add to this list based on their knowledge of the sexual complaints that abnormal genito-urinary anatomy, physiology, and infection engender. These include unexplainable pain and decreased sensation. There are also patients, some but not all of whom are conspicuously mentally ill, who compulsively insert objects into their pelvic orifices for mysterious reasons. I have seen two women who responded to different commonly used medications with disabling clitoral priapism. The mystery is what in their biochemical milieu could explain this frightening side effect.

A mental health professional is bound to encounter men and women who feel their genitals are abnormal, have changed coloration and appearance, or are misshapen either because the penis is too small or the labia minora are too large. Those who are looking for genital plastic surgery now have physicians who call themselves "aesthetic gynecologists." While some of these patients are thought to be displacing their social, interpersonal, and psychological concerns to their genitals, others may be unwilling to tell us what they are doing to their genitals during masturbation. These psychosomatic processes are not mysterious in the way others are, but they are often very difficult to modify. Without understanding the pathway to the symptom, any problem is more difficult to eradicate. Then there is the pathogenesis of problematic sexual function among some individuals with autism. I suspect that a large number of those who are described as being asexual in their orientation may be autistic. A socially inexperienced, friendless adult autistic patient whom I see in my practice portrays himself as a heterosexual "a-romantic," meaning he does not think he is capable of falling in love or of sustaining a loving relationship. Sex is something he can imagine; an intimate loving relationship is something he cannot. While most of the autistic patients whom I see do not have a regular sexual partner, the ones that do often have unusual symptom presentations, such as genital insensitivity or hypersensitivity. Teasing apart neural dysfunction from the effects of lack of ordinary attachment and socialization processes leaves me and others with a humble uncertainty.

From Painful Intercourse to Genito-Pelvic Pain/Penetration Disorder

This brings us to painful intercourse, a very common problem for women of all ages.[1] Physicians named the symptom *dyspareunia* centuries ago. They also recognized that some women had extreme difficulty tolerating a pelvic examination (not the typical apprehension) and often avoided the experience or became dramatically distraught during it. When such exams were medically necessary because of acute pelvic illness, these women could only be examined under anesthesia. When the physician could identify and treat the source of the pain, the symptom resolved. For example, infectious diseases were a recurring source.

In 1970 *vaginismus* was described as the state of prolonged spastic contraction of the circumvaginal muscles when digital or penile entry into the vagina was anticipated.[2] Partners found that penetration was mechanically difficult or impossible and that the vagina seemed to disappear. When intercourse was possible, it was often painful and terrifying. The woman's catastrophizing reactions to the imminence of penetration reduced the frequency of attempts and made it difficult for male partners to sustain an erection. (Vaginismus is occasionally encountered in lesbian women.) This led those couples who did not cease all sexual activity to restrict their behavior to manual or oral stimulation. Many of these couples only appeared for assistance when they desired to have a pregnancy.

A few years later *provoked vulvodynia* (or *vestibulodynia*) was described. A patient was given this diagnosis when she responded with pain to a light touch of her vulva with a cotton swab. Many of these women had no other apparent vestibular abnormalities. After years of assuming that unexplained dyspareunia, vaginismus, and the burning pain of vulvodynia were local genital pathologies, the idea began to emerge that perhaps the pelvis was the location of a central nervous system pain perception disorder. This idea was supported by an increased incidence of fibromyalgia, irritable bowel syndrome, and/or migraine headaches, and it focused greater clinical attention on women's pain. Clinicians began to notice that the perception of pain sometimes began before penetration actually began. Pain rightly skews medical and psychological interventions toward its relief. When the patient has other pelvic symptoms in addition to pain, as many women do, a careful urological/gynecological evaluation is required.

Every woman with dyspareunia should have a thorough pelvic examination and a careful differential diagnostic assessment. But when the woman has never been able to use tampons and is asymptomatic when penetration is not expected, the therapist can think of this as a penetration phobia. Some women with this dysfunction have regressed to the point that they cannot tolerate the knowledge of having an inner space. They do not like the idea that they have a vagina. This is hard to believe until you explore their concept of pelvic anatomy, which the woman does not like to visualize or consider. I have seen this among patients of all educational and socioeconomic levels.

In 2013, in DSM-5, dyspareunia was renamed *genito-pelvic pain/penetration disorder* to encompass the diverse aspects of this sexual dysfunction. About half of the women were noted to have developed the problem after a period of good sexual functioning; the others had had it from the beginning of their partner sexual activity. Genito-pelvic pain/penetration disorder is an excellent example of the interface of bodily problems, such as sensory abnormalities, low pain threshold, or recurrent vaginal infections, and psychosocial factors, both from early life and from their current relationship, that cause or enhance pain when penetration is greatly feared. This disorder can be used as a model for psychosomatic problems.

In clinics that specialize in treating this problem, psychologists, gynecologists, and physical therapists administer the treatments in coordination. Each discipline has found aspects of the problem to separately approach while working in a coordinated fashion. These teams develop theories about the fundamental nature of the problem. From the time that psychoanalytic professionals were viewed as experts in human sexuality, this problem was likely viewed as occurring at the interface of hysteria and frigidity. There was a time when investigations focused on pelvic mucosal hypersensitivity. The focus evolved to central pain perceptual disorder, with the observation that many of these women processed emotions about sex in very different ways. Today, although there is still an acknowledgment of the diverse pathways to the problem, greater emphasis is placed on interpersonal emotion regulation difficulties.[3] The field has accepted that any model to explain the phenomenon of genito-pelvic pain/penetration disorder must be complex. There is no single cause.

Outside specialized clinics, patients tend to receive only the treatments offered by the specialist they consult, often without ongoing coordination.

Many treatments have been employed, including use of progressive vaginal dilators, topical anesthetics, tricyclic antidepressants, corticosteroid creams, cognitive-behavioral therapy, couple's sex therapy, mindfulness therapy, biofeedback, pelvic floor relaxation, pain management, and vestibulectomy. Each modality has been demonstrated to help some women. There is no one approach that significantly helps most of these patients.

Similarities Between All Sexual Dysfunctions

All the sexual dysfunctions involve the perceiving brain, the reactive genitalia, the brain reacting to the genitalia, and the relationship situation in which sex is transacted. When a partner is involved, the partner's brain and genital function are also part of the complexity. Sexual dysfunctions are one of many forms of psychosomatic impairments. Do not assume, however, that specialists in psychosomatic medicine invariably consider sexual dysfunction to reside in their area of interest and competence. Almost all medical doctors have a group of patients who are thought to have psychosomatic problems that are difficult to resolve. Hypochondriasis comes to mind. Physicians are happy to refer these patients, but many of them are not interested in a referral and want to stay with their doctor. Given the high prevalence of dyspareunia, and the fact that many women do not seek medical or psychological help for painful intercourse,[4] it is likely that patients seeing you for other mental health issues may have a degree of this problem. Feel free to inquire when something makes you think about it. Sometimes you will learn of the dyspareunia from the patient's partner. This hidden pattern applies to all the sexual dysfunctions.

The interpersonal emotion regulation model has the advantage of illustrating the complexity of many dysfunctions.[3] I suspect that it even applies to male dysfunctions, particularly among older men. What seems to be different about genito-pelvic pain/penetration disorder is a body that announces, "I don't want to have intercourse," even as its owner is seeking assistance for her inability to have intercourse. I ask, "Why don't you want to have intercourse? "The answer, often, is, "Pain." "But why do you suppose you fear intercourse so?" The answer, often, is, "I don't know why I'm so terrified of it." "There is only one answer in this room that is not acceptable. It is, I don't know. I know you don't know with certainty, but please give me your best guess. You have been thinking about this for a long time." This line of questioning usually leads to productive discussion. Please feel free to borrow this method with any person with any dysfunction who claims ignorance.

I think about the patient's pain/penetration problem as another sexual dysfunction that is generated by a variety of complicated psychosomatic pathways. The woman has contradictory aims: she wants to be normal and be able to enjoy pain-free intercourse, yet she clearly would like to avoid it. She tells herself she has limited sexual desire, although sometimes this is true only for intercourse. Pain, especially in anticipation of intercourse, is a manifestation of her phobia. Recall that many men with psychogenic erectile dysfunction say they want to have intercourse but their penises are telling an opposite story. Contradictions are not confined to those with genito-pelvic pain/penetration disorder.

Suggestions for Treatment

I have some suggestions for you as you work with your first patients with this pelvic problem. Find an appropriate time to explain the psychological meaning of ambivalence to her. But be certain that she does not understand ambivalence to be a pathological state of being. Teach her that it is an ordinary normal psychological feeling toward many people and things in our lives—parents, siblings, lovers, husbands, and activities such as sexual behaviors. Do not assume that because the individual is highly educated, he or she understands ambivalence in this way and does not need such an explanation. Psychotherapy is a process of understanding mental life in general and the patient's mental processes in particular. I cannot separate the education that occurs during therapy from therapy's other processes, such as deepening trust of or the attachment to the therapist.

Second, in carefully listening to her talk about herself, ask yourself two basic questions about the pathway to her symptoms: 1) Is the patient not developmentally ready for sexual intercourse? 2) Does the patient not want to have sexual intercourse because of her assessment of her partner's character? Because these are not either/or possibilities, consider to what extent they both might be operative? The first question asks you to think about how a young girl who may not even be aware of her vaginal anatomy moves from this ordinary state of innocence to eagerness to try intercourse. What is known about the process? What are the intervening steps? What relationships, if any, are important? Mothers? Friends? Older sisters? Teachers? What other factors are involved? Tampons? Books and magazines? What adversities interfere with her development? Poor quality of parental bonding? Sexual and other forms of trauma? Personal serious physical illness?

As to the second question, it is difficult at any given time to understand the contribution of the patient's complaints about her partner in and outside the bedroom to her symptoms. The woman may want to believe that her complaints about her partner are of little actual importance. But over time this may become clearer to you and ultimately to her.

> The wife of a morbidly obese businessman, after years of phobic nonconsummation, chose artificial insemination to become pregnant. She had a lifelong phobia for penetration and panic-induced pain whenever they attempted to have intercourse. A number of therapists over many years failed to enable improvement. She and her husband gave up trying eventually. They continued in treatment to discuss other aspects of her life, including dilemmas she experienced dealing with her chronically depressed mother. Having dealt with both partners over a long period of time, I understood why she eventually characterized her husband as being a "vile, disgusting, crude, dishonest genius for making money." I had not seen her for 2 years after their divorce until she spotted me sitting at a large social gathering. She tapped me on the shoulder. When I stood up, she embraced me and with glee told me, "Guess what? I have a new boyfriend, and I love sexual intercourse and I have no pain. I am now normal! Thank you."

> An ambitious, high-striving, anxious college senior had an anxiety attack following her recent painless intercourse debut. She said it was clearly Catholic guilt. Her anxiety gradually lessened as she had more intercourse with the same man. They eventually parted ways, and she had a second boyfriend who, although handsome and charming, gave her pause because she was uncertain of his sincerity, stated ambitions, and work efforts. As her doubts increased, she began to have pain during intercourse. They worried because on two occasions they both had trouble locating her vaginal opening. With more attempts, the pain and presumed spasms disappeared. When asked how these improvements occurred, she gave two explanations. "My views of him have become more positive. I no longer think he doesn't have much of a future. Anyway, I think I am growing up. I feel more like a woman now."

I continue to wonder how we grow up. Which processes facilitate maturation? Which prevent it? How does maturation remodel us without our awareness? I believe the deeper goal of psychotherapy is to facilitate maturation, regardless of the ideology that informs the therapist. But how is this accomplished? I have my hunches, and you have some too and will likely acquire more as you accumulate clinical experience. These hunches coalesce into convictions that are difficult-to-impossible to test scientifically. But clinical work is far less scientific in its methods than it is humane in its goals.

A Frightening Thought

We clinicians do not trivialize the problem of genital pain. Not only does it take its toll on the woman's (and her partner's) sexual life, reproductive experiences, and a sense of personal adequacy, it may occasionally be the harbinger of something far more psychiatrically severe. Perhaps we should worry if the problem is the first form of a significant mental illness. I share this discomforting idea because I have had two patients among a dozen or so women with this pattern who have worked with me for a long time and whose lives eventually became far more tragic. I will tell you about just one of them.

> Carmen was unable to consummate her marriage of 20 years. She was a well-regarded teacher in the same school for 22 years. Her work there had been interrupted by a successful aortic valve replacement because of childhood rheumatic heart disease. She was a lively, expressive, physically active person who was fastidious about her appearance and proud that she did not look her age. She often brought up her conflicts between religion and sexual pleasure. She was her working husband's caregiver. "Poor Mike" was her frequent expression followed by an infectious laugh. She cared for him through his periodic months of self-doubt and persistent anxiety after the successful treatment of his testicular cancer. She ran the home and handled their finances and was particularly savvy about health insurance.
>
> I only had five sessions with her and Mike, who was quiet but vague when he spoke. Thereafter they were able to begin having painless intercourse. It seemed that discussion of her father's prancing around the house in his underwear and her witnessing his masturbation as an adolescent greatly frightened her.
>
> Carmen and a married sister did what they could for their socially isolated older sister, who had schizophrenia. Carmen described herself as having obsessive-compulsive disorder (OCD). I concurred and kept her on the high-dose selective serotonin reuptake inhibitor that she had been prescribed by another physician because it helped her with her obsessions about money and her compulsivity about work, home, and finances.
>
> After 10 years of once- or twice-a-month intercourse, sex seemed less important to the couple. She ceased being orgasmic on their increasingly rare painless intercourses. Then at age 57, after quitting the first job she held after retiring from teaching, she had the first of two psychotic depressions. She recovered from the first one but never had the confidence to return to the workplace. Three years later, shortly after the dose of an antipsychotic was lowered because of weight gain, she had a second episode from which her electroconvulsive therapy–induced recovery has been limited. She no longer is lively, her appearance has deteriorated, and she is remarkably quiet, repeating, "I am fine." She is not interested in doing anything around the house. She is 30 pounds heavier and does not like to move from her TV-watching chair. Mike is now retired. He is talkative and no longer vague. He manages every aspect of their lives and seems resigned to Carmen's new low level of functioning. He has accomplished this despite his own bout with significant physical illness that is likely the consequence of prior radiation treatment. Neither can remember when they last had sex. "I would like to, but Carmen is not the same woman."

Of course, I have no way of knowing whether Carmen and Mike's inability to consummate their marriage was related to her subsequent psychotic depression. I only can wonder whether her vaginal penetration phobia, which was so readily overcome, and her OCD, which was socially disguised through her energy, attention to organization and joy in handling details, and hovering care of "poor Mike," indicated a lifelong vulnerability that erupted into a florid psychotic state as she began to lose her youthful appearance. I have come to respect the possibility that this and most other sexual dysfunctions are still mysteries. While I have been able to help people with their sexual lives, I now realize that the gains made by patients from this valuable work do not guarantee their future health. With every dysfunction discussed in this book, we have seen that sexual life is embedded in other personal nonsexual matters. Patients like Carmen slap us into an awareness that we do not really know the nature of the underlying predispositions to dysfunction. We keep trying to understand.

References

1. van Lankveld JJ, Granot M, Weijmar Schultz WC, et al: Women's sexual pain disorders. J Sex Med 7(1, Pt 2):615–631, 2010
2. Masters WH, Johnson V: Human Sexual Inadequacy. Boston, MA, Little, Brown, 1970
3. Rosen NO, Bergeron S: Genito-pelvic pain through a dyadic lens: moving toward an interpersonal emotion regulation model of women's sexual dysfunction. J Sex Res 56(4–5):440–461, 2019
4. Harlow BL, Kunitz GG, Nguyen RH, et al: The prevalence of the symptom consistent with the diagnosis of vulvodynia: population-based estimates from 2 geographical regions. Am J Obstet Gynecol 210(1):40.e1-8, 2014

10 | Your Professional Development

Making Distinctions

Mental health professionals make distinctions, not only for the purposes of initially diagnosing our patients but also in our everyday work with them. We educate, motivate, and support our patients in their quest to do better in life, in or outside the bedroom, through these distinctions. Some distinctions we make are simple, such as distinguishing between a sexual function and a sexual identity problem. Others are subtle, such as highlighting the differences between apology, regret, and remorse; distinguishing disagreement from argument; and clarifying with a couple that they possess two different subjective marriages. Some distinctions are harder to classify. We may point out that the aesthetic appreciation of beauty is not the same as sexual desire for the beautiful person. Some require extensive explanation, for instance, to clarify the differences between a problem, a dilemma, and a conundrum.

The differences between a problem, a dilemma, and a conundrum introduce professionals and their patients into certain realities beyond DSM-5 sexual diagnoses. Patients seek our assistance for a sexual problem that they recognize they cannot solve. Lifelong premature ejaculation and women's anorgasmia, for example, are problems that we may be able to help patients to overcome. The man can be assisted to provide a longer, more sensuous duration of intercourse for himself and his partner. The woman can be helped to discover her orgasmic capacity in solo and partnered situations. And when a couple's sexual lives are characterized by both of these patterns, as many young peoples' lives are, the professional can be instrumental in helping both feel normal about their new sexual capacities and more optimistic about their union. Problem solved, perhaps not quickly, but overcome nonetheless without any negative effects.

I think of a dilemma as a problem whose solution carries with it a significant, often permanent negative consequence. After an extramarital love affair, for instance, the couple can survive and emotionally prosper in multiple dimensions of their lives, but each of them will be psychologically changed. They both remain aware of the affair for years to come, whether they speak of it or not. Each may have lingering mood changes and vivid memories each time he or she encounters any references to infidelity, which, of course, abound in the news, television, and movies. It is part of the continuing dilemma of past experiences. Some couples bear a more serious version of continuing problem when all sexual behaviors between them permanently cease after apparently moving beyond the crisis of betrayal. Another example of a dilemma occurs when an adolescent declares a new trans identity. Parents are typically uncertain and continuously ambivalent about whether the trans aspiration is a wise or a foolish new sense of reality. Some parents disagree with each other, with the difference of opinion leading to increasing marital friction, or the father disengages from the teenager while the mother supports the aspiration, fearing the child's suicide. Each parent, however, fears condemning the youngster to an unhappy future. For the adolescent the new trans status may painfully shift peer relationships and social, sexual, and other developmental processes. The person can start life exploring a gender change via binary or nonbinary adaptations, but not without significant costs. These costs become apparent whether we are seeing the teenager alone, the parents alone, or the family together. Seemingly successful transition, even among the famous, is not without costs that must be borne.

A conundrum is a dilemma whose solution may bring on a situation as bad as the original problem. Here are a few examples.

1. A man has a "fling with stripper for a while," which costs him thousands of dollars in support of her various frequent financial needs, only to discover she is pregnant with his child. When the child is born, it is apparent to him and his wife, who has been told about his new predicament, that the woman is a grossly inadequate mother. The man, his wife, and the baby's mother each have a conundrum.

2. After a couple begins an agreed-on quest for a child through fertility treatment, the couple's sexual pleasures disappear. They were led to expect a little of this by their physician. Now, after three in vitro fertilization (IVF) failures and tens of thousands of dollars, the husband feels he is hostage to his spouse's "obsessive" need for a baby. Never one to express his conflicted feelings and not wanting to further upset her, he finds a new sexual partner, who after 4 months begins to pressure him to leave his wife. He refuses a fourth IVF attempt and separates from his wife. Within 2 weeks, his wife, who became too depressed to go to work, attempts suicide. He re-

turns home to care for her, which provokes rage in his heavily drinking paramour, who begs him to return.

3. A successful businessman 16 years younger than his 53-year-old girlfriend has never been able to have sexual desire for anyone he loves. His love-lust split has kept him single and anxious. He is a charming, intelligent, charismatic man, but as treatment planning focuses on discussing the origins of the problematic pattern, he says, "I want the past to be the past—I don't think I can talk about it. I love her, I want to make love with her, but I really don't." She adds, "He told me he found the female genitals disgusting; once he touched my breasts, but he was too uncomfortable for me to enjoy it. He just wants to cuddle while clothed." We finish the session discussing an asexual life together, when his girlfriend adds that he has engaged several of her friends or colleagues in providing oral sex for him. "How am I to handle that socially?"

While we try to assist patients when they are trapped by a conundrum, many ask for our advice. I think our best counsel is to define their situation as a conundrum, which means there are no painless solutions. Each decision will yield a new significant moral, psychological, economic, or interpersonal problem. We must be careful not to think we know what the patient ought to do. We can only help our patients consider the options and their consequences and focus on what they are going through affectively.

Their conundrum helps us to counsel future patients with dilemmas to avoid decisions that may create a conundrum. When a patient says about some personal dilemma, "At least it can't get any worse," I usually pop up with, "Yes, it can!" Teaching about conundrums can be a major contribution to their lives. Diagnoses, per se, do not lead to divorce or psychological deterioration, but conundrums often do.

Helping the Patient Live a Better Life

Our task to help the patient to live a better life is a lofty goal. It is sometimes attainable, but it is easy to lose sight of the goal because of our seeming first responsibility to eradicate or attenuate the patients' symptoms. Primary care doctors hear about symptoms of anxiety and depression daily and are the major source of prescriptions for benzodiazepines and antidepressants. When we focus on clinical sexual problems, we have a clearer window into the circumstances that our patient is facing. We must be careful that our education and our belief in some ideology do not blind us to our patients' actual realities. Some therapists are educated in a medical model of managing problems with an emphasis on their biological contributions and treatments.[1] Others are trained in cognitive-behavioral therapy and are eager to apply their means of attenuating these symptoms. I have no arguments with our collective toolbox, but in this book I have stressed development, adversity, and trauma rather than the brain changes that these early life experiences are known to create or the therapy techniques that are popular today.

As emphasized in earlier chapters, the cause of a problem need not be reduced to a single factor. In fact, for most problems that have been carefully studied, influences have been found to include biology, past experience, current psychological circumstances, interpersonal relationships, and culture.[2,3] My advice to a young professional is to respect what you know, but recognize that your knowledge is incomplete. This is not your personal deficiency. While you can learn more, you cannot remove all the mystery. This awareness prevents arrogance, which is often quite destructive to a patient's recovery and growth because it is an oversimplification of the patient's life. It is my hope that understanding the distinctions between an uncomplicated problem, a dilemma, and a conundrum will prevent superficial responses to complicated circumstances. The goal of leading a better life seems useful, even when we cannot quite get there. Patients have certainly valued our efforts.

Understanding That Psychotherapy Is Now a Generic Term

Psychotherapy is an umbrella term under which a vast array of differing interventions exists.[4] Its hundreds of forms are supported by different ideologies and vocabularies. No one brand of psychotherapy is applicable to everything that ails humans. A professional's preferred form of psychotherapy, based on education and indoctrination during the period of formal training, generates a personal identity that carries with it a belief in the superiority of what has been taught to them. It also creates affiliation patterns with others who share similar beliefs. Despite literally thousands of studies, superiority has not been consistently demonstrated for any one form of psychotherapy. This, too, can keep us humble.

Psychotherapy is a purposeful, professional, intimate conversational process that focuses on the patient's subjective, interpersonal, developmental, and biological life in order to benefit the patient. Psychotherapy has rules for its conduct, concepts about its processes, and ethical obligations. Many psychotherapies rest on an assumption that emotional growth and symptom relief are mediated through relationships.[5] Ultimately, faith in the importance of the therapeutic relationship is required. Insight has been shown to have a moderate correlation with outcome across diagnostic categories and across schools of thought.[6] Patients indirectly express their faith that the relationship with the therapist is vital by participating in psychotherapy or by showing disappointment when they receive a treatment other than psychotherapy from a psychiatrist or a nurse practitioner who only prescribes medication. Those who seek our assistance do not all share this assumption, however. Disbelievers (and, at times, some believers) may want something else at a particular time. This could be a web-based program, medication, or hospitalization. Or they may be looking for agreement with their position in a conflict, want to be found competent to continue administering their affairs, be seeking an accommodation for test taking, and so forth. As patients and therapists share a psychotherapy process, they come to believe that the alliance between them is crucial to the process.[7]

In discussing the ordinary complexities of sexual dysfunction and sexual identity concerns, I have not recommended a particular type of psychotherapy to use in providing care. This is because therapy is a unique experience based on the characteristics of each patient or couple. You provide an emerging understanding of the patient's feelings, conflicts, and dilemmas through your individual style of helping the patient identify and process them. These two characteristics of the therapist—the quest to understand and your inevitably distinctive style—plus the uniqueness of each patient, are far more important than the theory you may believe in. In seeking to understand the complaint, we look for its precipitants, for the forces that maintain it, and for predisposing vulnerabilities. After a half century of defining sexual problems, the field has moved beyond recommending one brand of therapy. Today, a sex therapist is someone willing to directly consider these issues; he or she is not a person with one method of treatment.

Recognizing Commonalities of Psychotherapy and Love

Well-managed psychotherapy resembles love in certain ways. The therapist does not literally love the patient. But the therapist is likely to experience most of the elements of love during their relationship, although at a much lesser intensity than in early adult-adult love relationships. We feel interest in, pleasure in being with, and appreciation of the patient. We care about and try to promote the welfare of the patient, and we maintain the belief that the patient is likely to be better off with us than without us.[8] These are most of the characteristics of love relationships. What we do not have, and do not desire to have, is the ambition to express our erotic and sexual selves with the patient. We provide psychological intimacy, we demonstrate a form of commitment, and, while our personal revelations are few, we foster a special kind of friendship. We are not friends in the ordinary sense of a two-way process. We do not socialize together. But what we contribute to the patient's life induces him or her to affectionately regard and highly appreciate us. The word we use to describe the type of person who is skillful at this one-way friendship is *psychotherapist*.

This idea is important because the ingredients of love realized in a psychotherapeutic relationship facilitate maturation. This should not come as a surprise, since parents' relationships to their children are also characterized by interest, pleasure, appreciation, devotion, and the conviction that their offspring needs them in their lives. I do not want to overemphasize this similarity. I just want to draw your attention to it. Most relationships with mental health professionals last less than six visits.[9] In short-term work, the comparison may be irrelevant. But in longer relationships the analogy speaks to a central question of how therapy works.[10]

Ensuring Role Satisfaction

When young professionals are looking for a job in an institution, they must be careful to evaluate whether the role they are considering will provide them with an opportunity to conduct psychotherapy. Many institutions will respond to your inquiry with "of course" because they consider patient care and psychotherapy to be one and the same. It is reasonable of you to ask about expectations for productivity, time per visit, frequency of permitted visits, and specific programs you will be a part of. Please recognize that institutions need to make a bit of a profit on your work. They consider your economic cost to them—salary plus benefits and start-up inefficiencies—when evaluating the economic viability of your position. You, the institution, and the patient can each benefit from structuring your work for psychotherapy. Consider it your responsibility to evaluate the culture of the institution—that is, their traditions of providing mental health services.

Job satisfaction is very important to your professional development. If your work is not structured correctly, you may not be able to deal with patients' psychological challenges, let alone their sexual concerns. Job dissatisfaction robs you of the pleasure of continuing professional development. I prefer to think of professional life as a career rather than a job. This distinction has to do with maintaining a commitment to personal growth rather than to simply managing patients. Professional growth comes from dealing with patients, of course, but institutional demands and policy changes can make therapists unhappy. Some professionals then work only for the income; others concentrate on finding a new position. I have seen many professionals who are deprived of the pleasures inherent in professional maturation. Burnout is much written about lately.[11]

Returning to the Questions in Chapter One

Do We Know Something That Observant Laypersons Do Not Know?

Well, there are some brilliant laypersons in the world. Much of what all of us know about life processes and sexuality can be found in fiction. Fiction illustrates what professionals struggle to articulate. The descriptions of infidelity in *Anna Karenina* or *Madame Bovary* are far more comprehensive, compelling, and educational than, say, Chapter 6 of this book. But in terms of everyday sexual concerns as they present to us, the answer to this question is, "Yes." Our ability to gain the trust of patients to share their privacy with us teaches us things that others may only generally know. We learn about sexuality in its highly individual manner. This education enables us to help others in a way that laypersons cannot.

Do We Have Esoteric Information or a Frame of Understanding That Is More or Less Unique to Us?

I think we do. The esoteric includes the range of gender diversities, the even greater range of paraphilia, and the uniqueness of individuals' well-hidden sexual identity mosaics. Our unique frames of reference include knowledge of innumerable ways people can mentally suffer; how this suffering relates to past events and processes; how interpersonal relationships evolve in the privacy of a couple's life; and the continuous role of development throughout the life cycle. When we read media accounts of a person's sexuality, we realize that there is always more to the story. By realizing the complexity of our patients' sexualities, we provide respect for their struggles required to overcome problematic patterns.

To What Extent Can Clinical Science Help Us?

I would like to answer this question with a resounding, "To a very large extent." But I am not certain. Many aspects of clinical science have advanced our work considerably, particularly in the realm of medications and HIV. Much of it demonstrates the useful insight that a previous assumption is not correct. It is perhaps because I am so struck by the patients I cannot help, that I am skeptical. I read or review a large number of papers per year about clinical sexuality and am often disappointed with how the ideas, supported by statistically significant P values, do not help me with the dilemmas that I am called on to face in treatment. Clinical science selects subjects to study on the basis of meeting criteria for a diagnosis, whereas I am called upon to take care of individuals who have that diagnosis but who present with unique dilemmas. Science obscures the uniqueness of the research subjects through large sample sizes. I relate to their uniqueness. Nonetheless, many of clinical science's findings form the background for a future breakthrough. Although I am a believer in clinical science, it is an inefficient, frustrating process for clinicians. The next question is a slight rephrasing of this one.

Is the Knowledge Generated by Clinical Science Useful to the Process of Helping?

Occasionally, it provides a tool. Sildenafil, a great medical advance brought to clinicians in 1998, has helped many, but it also has failed many. Mindfulness as a therapeutic approach helps some women reacquaint themselves with sexual desire. I greatly respect the work that goes into clinical studies, but I fear that science cannot even measure the variables that shape human contradictions and paradoxes. Much sexological science that aims to help clinicians actually helps the researchers to learn about scientific methods and their limitations. As many point out, correlation is not the same as causality. My belief is that both professional developmental processes that come from immersion in clinical work and findings from published studies enable us to appreciate patients' private dilemmas. Sexuality provides a clear lens through which to view the subject of mental health, although many sexological studies focus on sexual and not mental health. I strongly believe that following the trends in clinical sexological science provides clinicians with an avenue of personal focus and growth. It also helps us from becoming too dogmatic or authoritative because we know that it is far easier to have a conviction than to prove it to be correct. All of us are likely to be wrong at times. My answer is, "Yes, clinical science occasionally changes our assumptions, but it more often is a force that keeps us humble."

Emphasizing Professional Development

In my professional setting, where differently trained mental health professionals come as staff members, clinical rotators, fellows, and conference attendees to share twice-weekly case conferences, many of us have noticed that ideologically informed professionals gradually lose their allegiance to their schools of thought. This happens slowly as they use their framework to explain the patient's problem. At best, their models explain an aspect of the patient's symptoms. Psychoanalysts, behavioral therapists, and biological psychiatrists, for example, begin with very different explanatory concepts and notions about what should be done to help the patient. When they arrive at our setting, few seem to be able to articulate the patient's dilemmas, contradictions, paradoxes, character traits, or social conflicts that they are currently facing. They emphasize diagnosis and symptoms rather than the person whose life qualified for the diagnosis. But over time, as individual patients and couple's actual circumstances are appreciated, the passion for their ideological model attenuates. Therapists typically still prefer the language of their ideology and maintain the professional identity they trained in, but they are less fervent. Accumulating clinical experience accompanied by peer discussions changes perceptions of patients' realities and leads to a more realistic assessment of therapy goals. It also begins to shape the presenter's view of identifying information. Instead of "This is a 45-year-old divorced woman complaining of anxiety and depression," we tend to be introduced to a 45-year-old unemployed divorced Caucasian mother of 6- and 8-year-old daughters, a recent community college graduate, who is depressed and having panic experiences following the death of her mother. This improved description of the patient helps all of us in the conference to better appreciate who the patient is. When we begin to hear of the patient's sexual concerns, we have an ever better context to understand him or her.

Judging from the preponderance of papers in psychiatric journals during the last two decades that focus on the brain and its changes with psychiatric disorders, academic psychiatry has tilted toward an emphasis on diagnosis, medication management, and evidence-based interventions. Many psychiatry residents are trained with this emphasis. This training has a limited utility when it comes to understanding and treating sexual identity, sexual function, and interpersonal relationship concerns in psychotherapy. It is, however, a wonderful background for beginning to understand clinical sexual matters. The shift in psychiatry away from psychotherapy has opened the door for other mental health professionals to pay attention to sexual concerns and their amelioration. This is an excellent opportunity to develop a niche specialty that will be greatly appreciated in your community, as professionals who are known to be knowledgeable and interested in clinical sexuality are few and far between. I would like psychiatrists to be interested in, and gain experience with, clinical sexuality. After all, even patients with serious psychiatric disorders have a sexual life. There is reason to believe that their sexual lives are more fraught than the sexual lives of mentally healthier individuals.[12] More importantly, I think interest in patients' sexuality can facilitate patient and professional maturation.

Eventually most mental health professionals come to realize that they are in the life-cycle business in that their patients are in different life phases that each carry unique sensibilities and vulnerabilities. It is as though there are seasons to a person's life with separate sexual possibilities and liabilities. We can be of assistance to patients in every era of their lives, but what we do and how we do it vary considerably.

Clinicians also come to appreciate how an illness in one family member brings considerable burdens to others. I wonder why these ideas are not introduced at the beginning of all mental health training. Early professional education teaches students how to conduct its favored brand or brands of psychotherapy. Many therapists have no experience with couples or families or even with talking to them, claiming federal rules of confidentiality. Such rigid rules ignore the interrelatedness of people and the numerous ways life can be improved. Professional maturation is characterized by flexibility and change rather than purity of method.

When I began in the field of clinical sexuality, any credentialed professional interested in sexual problems was a welcomed novel addition to the community. Even much older individuals and couples came to see me. Over time I sensed, however, that the majority of my patients were within 15 years of my age. In my 40s I began frequently hearing about infidelity for the first time. Now that I am a senior professional, I am seeing many more people who are also seniors, not just for sexual concerns. What this now affords me is a view of how many patients no longer have a sexual life; some have basically never had much of one.

In taking care of young people, one works to free them from their internal or external constraints so that they can have more personal and interpersonal freedom, including the freedom to enjoy their bodies in sexual expression. Taking care of older patients, however, alerts us to the fact that prior processes—betrayals, diaper fetishes, abandonment of children, vocational inadequacy, sexual abuse, serious physical illness, and so forth—have consequences. We try to lessen the burden from these matters. Sometimes, we only commiserate with their lost opportunities.

Melvin, a retired pharmaceutical salesman with Tourette's syndrome associated with his obsessive-compulsive personality, comes to see me because of crying spells and suicidal ideation. His symptoms quickly improve with an antidepressant and several conversations during which he explained that his father's inability to earn enough money had remained with Melvin all of his life. Melvin's family had moved at least three times in the night to avoid eviction. This humiliated him and motivated him to never be poor. He worked from age 13 onward and put himself through college. His rise to the upper middle class was accompanied by a constant worry about whether the doctors he routinely called on liked him. This anxiety persisted during the two decades when he was the one of the best salesmen in the nation for his company. His anxiety about being liked by doctors dominated conversations with his wife, Marjorie. Now that he no longer works, Marjorie becomes irritated with him when he expresses the same anxiety about their friends. At our second session he says he has been crying recently over his recognition that his preoccupation with work has prevented him from having a sex life with Marjorie. "I was always too nervous. We had sex regularly for a few months, but only until Marjorie became pregnant with our only child. I have disappointed myself that I avoided sex for the last 30+ years."

Patient stories are different from one person or one couple to the next. So many, however, tell of years of "loving each other" but lacking sexual behavior together. Sex is highly desired but is too frightening to participate in for many adults. You will be seeing people like Melvin and his wife when they are much younger. As you are relatively young, many of your patients will be at the stage in their lives when helping them to free themselves from their internal constraints and helping them to articulate their external barriers to enjoying their lives more are the relevant clinical tasks. It is my hope that you can prevent some of the sad outcomes like the one that Melvin and Marjorie experienced. I think this is a worthy endeavor. I hope you do, too.

References

1. Berlin FS: A conceptual overview and commentary on gender dysphoria. J Am Acad Psychiatry Law 44(2):246–252, 2016
2. Lewis M: Brain change in addiction as learning, not disease. N Engl J Med 379(16):1551–1560, 2018
3. Rosen NO, Bergeron S: Genito-pelvic pain through a dyadic lens: moving toward an interpersonal emotion regulation model of women's sexual dysfunction. J Sex Res 56(4–5):440–461, 2019
4. Høgland P: Insight into insight psychotherapy (editorial). Am J Psychiatry 175(10):923–924, 2018
5. Horvath AO, Del Re AC, Flückiger C, Symonds D: Alliance in individual psychotherapy. Psychotherapy (Chic) 48)(1):9–16, 2011
6. Jamieson S, Huber J, Ehrenthal JC, et al: Association between insight and outcome of psychotherapy: systematic review and meta-analysis. Am J Psychiatry 175(10):961–969, 2018
7. Høgland P: Exploration of the patient-therapist relationship in psychotherapy. Am J Psychiatry 171:1056–1066, 2014
8. Levine SB: Love and therapy, in Barriers to Loving: A Clinician's Perspective. New York, Routledge, 2014, pp 109–123
9. Barrett MS, Chau W, Crits-Christoph P, et al: Early withdrawal from mental health treatment: implications for psychotherapy practice. Psychotherapy: Theory, Research, Practice, Training 45(2):247–267, 2008
10. Kazdin AE: Mediators and mechanisms of change in psychotherapy. Annu Rev Clin Psychol 3:1–27, 2007

11. Volpe U, Luciano M, Palumbo C, et al: Risk of burnout among early career mental health professionals. J Psychiatr Ment Health Nurs 21(9):774–781, 2014

12. Kockott G, Pfeiffer W: Sexual disorders in nonacute psychiatric patients. Compr Psychiatry 37(1):56–61, 1996

Appendix

Further Reading and Resources

Recent General Textbooks on Care of Sexual Problems

Binik YM, Hall KSK (eds): Principles and Practices of Sex Therapy, 5th Edition. New York, Guilford, 2014

Goldstein I, Clayton AH, Goldstein AT, et al (eds): Textbook of Female Function and Dysfunction: Diagnosis and Treatment. New York, Wiley, 2018

Hertlein KM, Weeks GR, Gambescia N (eds): Systemic Sex Therapy, 2nd Edition. New York, Routledge, 2015

IsHak WW (ed): The Textbook of Clinical Sexual Medicine. Springer International Publishing, 2017

Levine SB, Risen CB, Althof SE (eds): Handbook of Clinical Sexuality for Mental Health Professionals, 3rd Edition. New York, Routledge, 2016

Selected Journals Devoted to Human Sexuality

AIDS
Archives of Sexual Behavior
Fertility and Sterility
Human Reproduction
Journal of Sex and Marital Therapy
Journal of Sex Research
Journal of Sexual Medicine
Journal of Women's Health
LGBT Health
Psychoneuroendocrinology

Academic Databases and Search Engines

Cochrane Library (subscription required)
Current Contents (subscription required)
Google Scholar (free)
MedlinePlus (free)
PsychINFO (subscription required)
Psychology's Feminist Voices (free)
PubMed (free)
PubPsych (free)

Major Sexology Organizations

AASECT: American Association of Sexuality Educators, Counselors and
  Therapists
Canadian Sex Research Forum (CSRF)
ESSM: European Society for Sexual Medicine
IASR: International Academy of Sex Research
ISSWSH: International Society for the Study of Women's Sexual Health
Kinsey Institute
Society of Australian Sexologists (SAS)
Society for Sex Therapy and Research (SSTAR)
Society for the Scientific Study of Sexuality (SSSS)
WPATH: World Professional Association for Transgender Health

Index

Page numbers printed in **boldface** type refer to tables or figures.